# CANADA: LIVING WITH RADIATION

 Atomic Energy Control Board    Commission de contrôle de l'énergie atomique    Canada

**Canadian Cataloguing in Publication Data**

Main entry under title:

Canada: Living with Radiation

Issued also in French under title:
Canada : Vivre avec le rayonnement
Includes bibliographical references.
ISBN 0-660-16036-6
Cat. no. CC172-7/1995E

1. Radiation -- Health aspects.
2. Radiation -- Safety measures.
I. Canada. Atomic Energy Control Board.
II. Canadian Nuclear Services.
III. Title : Canada : Living with Radiation.

QC475.C32 1995  363.17'99  C95-980086-7

Available in Canada through

your local bookseller

or by mail from

Canada Communication Group-Publishing
Ottawa, Canada  K1A 0S9

Cat. no. CC172-7/1995E
ISBN 0-660-16036-6

*Également disponible en français*

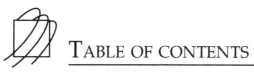

# TABLE OF CONTENTS

# LIST OF FIGURES

## ACKNOWLEDGEMENTS

This document was inspired in part by the informative booklet *Living with Radiation* produced by the National Radiological Protection Board of the United Kingdom. The Atomic Energy Control Board of Canada is grateful for permission from the NRPB to imitate that publication and borrow sections from it.

*Canada: Living with Radiation* was prepared for the Atomic Energy Control Board by Canadian Nuclear Services, 1400 Bayly Street, Office Mall 2, Suite 10, Pickering, Ontario, L1W 3R2. The authors were Dr. David Myers of Pembroke, Ontario, Dr. Peter Barry of Deep River, Ontario, and Mr. Robert Wilson of West Hill, Ontario, who also was editor. The assistance, in reviewing the document, of Mr. David McMillan, Head of the Chemistry Department, and students Courtney Armstrong, Rob Bennet, Mark Johannsen and Mary Anne Rogers, all of Sir Oliver Mowat Collegiate, Scarborough, Ontario, is gratefully acknowledged.

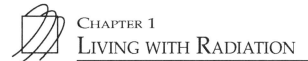

# CHAPTER 1
# LIVING WITH RADIATION

Canadians are exposed daily to a variety of naturally occurring radiation. Heat and light from the sun, essential for life, are familiar examples. The sun, like other stars, is also the source of other types of radiation which are not detectable by the human senses. Radium and uranium are naturally occurring materials which have been found to emit radiation and so have been called *radioactive*. There are also various types of artificially produced forms of radiation that are employed routinely in modern living, such as radio and television waves and microwaves. X-rays, another common type of radiation, are widely used in medicine as are some man-made radioactive substances. These emit radiation just like naturally occurring radioactive materials.

Based on the effects they produce in matter, two classes of radiation, *ionizing* and *non-ionizing*, have been defined. Ionizing radiation which is fully described in Chapter 2 includes x-rays and the various types of radiation emitted by radioactive materials. Non-ionizing radiation includes heat or infrared radiation, visible light, ultraviolet light, radio and radar waves (Figure 1.1). All radiation appears to have harmful biological effects if its intensity is sufficiently high.

## BENEFITS AND RISKS OF RADIATION

The benefits of naturally occurring non-ionizing radiation are obvious to us all. There would be no life on earth without the heat and light received as radiation from the sun.

Both ionizing and non-ionizing radiation are now produced artificially in many forms and their beneficial uses are widespread. Man-made, non-ionizing radiation is the basis of modern communication systems; it is employed to make our streets safer at night, and throughout industry in modern processes for construction (lasers) and chemical analysis. Artificially produced ionizing radiation is widely employed in medicine for the diagnosis and treatment of tumours, in industry for level measurement and for quality control of welding, in sterilization of medical equipment, and even for eradicating certain insect pests.

Ionizing radiation must be employed with care. Soon after x-rays were discovered in the late 19th century, harmful effects of ionizing radiation were observed. As with all other types of radiation, exposures to ionizing radiation must be carefully controlled in practice so that we may realize the benefits without experiencing harmful effects.

The most serious harmful effect of exposure to natural or man-made ionizing radiation that may be expected at the levels of exposure in modern usage, is a slight increase in cancers and possibly inherited defects in exposed groups. Not all exposed persons or their offspring will experience these effects but there will be an increased chance they will occur. For example, in an unexposed group the cancer rate may be 26% over a lifetime, and in an exposed population it may be 27%.

To realize the benefits of ionizing radiation without experiencing serious levels of harm is a challenge. Careful control of the source of radiation and the levels of exposure is required. Practices which have marginal benefits but cause significant exposure should not be permitted or should be discontinued if they are being practiced. An example of this was the use of x-ray machines in shoe stores to see if a shoe fitted. These are no longer in use as the benefit did not warrant the potential risk from the radiation exposure.

| SOME BENEFICIAL APPLICATIONS OF RADIATION | |
|---|---|
| **Ionizing** | **Non-Ionizing** |
| Medical Diagnoses | Radio |
| Cancer Treatment | Television |
| Density & Level Measurement | Radar |
| Weld Inspection | Microwave Communication |
| Sterilization of Medical Items | Microwave Cooking |
| Control of Certain Insects | Heating (Infra-red) |
| Food Preservation | Lighting |
| Safety Devices (smoke detectors) | Laser Surgery, etc. |

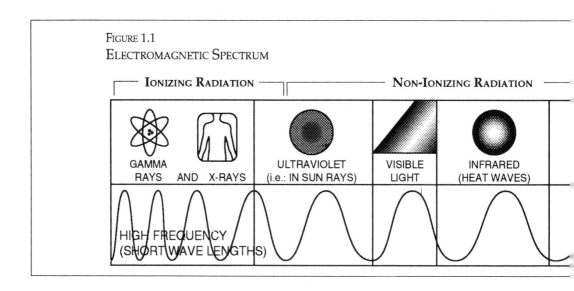

FIGURE 1.1
ELECTROMAGNETIC SPECTRUM

⌐ IONIZING RADIATION ⌐ NON-IONIZING RADIATION ⌐

GAMMA RAYS AND X-RAYS | ULTRAVIOLET (i.e.: IN SUN RAYS) | VISIBLE LIGHT | INFRARED (HEAT WAVES)

HIGH FREQUENCY (SHORT WAVE LENGTHS)

## Public Concern and Perception of Risk

Surveys have shown that many people have a poor understanding of the risks associated with the activities of modern living. For example, some people will not take an air flight, because they perceive it to be unsafe, but they will drive in an automobile without concern; yet the risk per kilometre of a fatality from flying on a commercial airline is much less than for driving, in Canada.

Exposure to ionizing radiation from radioactive materials is also considered by many persons to have a high risk. This could be due to the association of ionizing radiation with nuclear weapons, or because ionizing radiation is mysterious and like most types of radiation, other than heat and light, cannot be sensed. It could also be because it may cause cancer, a disease many people consider particularly dreadful. Whatever the reason, there is a fear of ionizing radiation. This booklet attempts to inform readers about ionizing radiation, its uses and the risks associated with it, and to put these risks in perspective with the risks of other activities and practices.

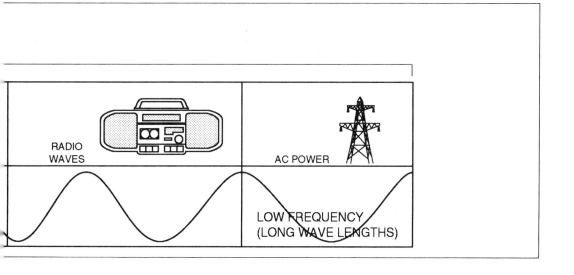

RADIO WAVES

AC POWER

LOW FREQUENCY
(LONG WAVE LENGTHS)

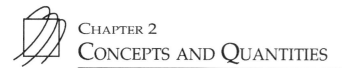

CHAPTER 2
# CONCEPTS AND QUANTITIES

## RADIOACTIVITY AND THE MAKEUP OF MATTER

Humans have always lived in the presence of low levels of ionizing radiation, although this fact was not known until late in the 19th century. Ionizing radiation in the form of x-rays was first discovered in 1895, while natural radioactivity was discovered in 1896. The universe, earth, and even our own bodies are now known to be naturally radioactive. The small amounts of natural radioactivity that are present in our bodies do not appear to be of any benefit to us, but are simply the consequences of the natural radioactivity of the earth and the rest of the universe. The heat of the earth's core, which is responsible for natural phenomena such as volcanoes, hot springs, continental drift and the formation of mountain ranges, depends largely on its natural radioactivity.

To understand natural radioactivity, it is useful to know something about the basic makeup of matter. Matter is composed of *elements:* the most common elements in our own bodies are hydrogen, carbon, nitrogen, oxygen, sodium, potassium, calcium, chlorine and phosphorus.

Elements consist of characteristic *atoms,* which have a very small core called a *nucleus* and from one to about 100 even smaller *electrons.* These circle in orbit about the nucleus in much the same manner as the earth and other planets circle the sun.

The simplest atom is hydrogen. It consists of a nucleus containing one positively-charged particle called a *proton* which is orbited by one negatively-charged electron. The positive and negative charges are in balance, so the atom is electrically neutral.

This most common form of hydrogen is abundant in nature and is designated hydrogen-1, where the number 1 refers to the relative mass of the nucleus. Hydrogen also exists in nature in small amounts as hydrogen-2 or deuterium (Figure 2.1). The nucleus of deuterium is twice as heavy as that of hydrogen-1 and consists of one proton, plus a neutral particle of equal mass called a *neutron.* The chemical properties of an element depend on the number of protons in the nucleus and the equivalent number of electrons orbiting the nucleus; thus deuterium behaves chemically in the same manner as hydrogen-1. Both hydrogen-1 and

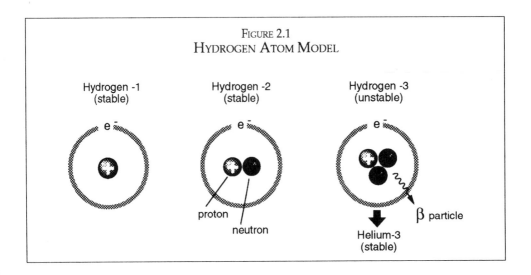

FIGURE 2.1
HYDROGEN ATOM MODEL

Hydrogen -1
(stable)

Hydrogen -2
(stable)

Hydrogen -3
(unstable)

e⁻

e⁻

e⁻

proton

neutron

β particle

Helium-3
(stable)

deuterium are *stable* atoms which emit no radiation.

A third variety of hydrogen that exists in nature in even smaller amounts than deuterium is hydrogen-3 or tritium. The tritium nucleus is three times as heavy as that of hydrogen-1 and consists of one proton plus two neutrons. Its chemical properties are again similar to those of hydrogen-1. The imbalance of protons and neutrons in the tritium nucleus leads to a natural tendency for this nucleus to rearrange its structure; that is to say, the tritium nucleus is *unstable*. A small, negatively charged electron called a *beta particle* is ejected at high speed from one of the neutrons. The effect is the conversion of this neutron into a proton and the transformation of the hydrogen-3 into another element called helium-3, which happens to be a stable atom.

This is one of the simplest examples of natural radioactivity. The natural tendency of a radioactive atom, or *radionu-*

*clide*, to rearrange itself is characteristic of the radionuclide and is measured by its *half-life*. This is the time taken for half the original number of radioactive atoms to decay into another type of atom, emitting radiation in the process. After one half-life, the amount of radionuclide is reduced to one-half, after two half-lives to

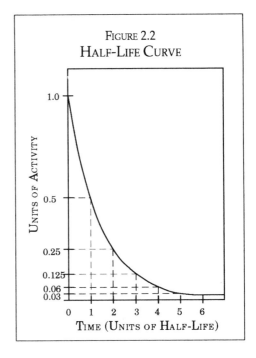

FIGURE 2.2
HALF-LIFE CURVE

UNITS OF ACTIVITY

1.0

0.5

0.25

0.125

0.06
0.03

0    1    2    3    4    5    6

TIME (UNITS OF HALF-LIFE)

one-quarter, after three half-lives to one eighth, and so on (Figure 2.2). The half-life of tritium is about 12 years. Thus any tritium formed centuries ago would have disappeared or decayed to negligible levels by now.

There is a natural concentration of tritium in our environment. This is the result of its formation in the upper atmosphere by the action of *cosmic rays* from outer space. Natural tritium is thus called a *cosmogenic* radionuclide. Another important cosmogenic radionuclide is carbon-14.

Some radionuclides have formed part of the material of the earth ever since the earth was first formed about five billion years ago. These are called *primordial* radionuclides and include potassium-40, thorium-232 and uranium-238. As before, the number corresponds to the weight of the nucleus. This weight is relative to the weight of a proton or a neutron each of which is assigned a weight of one (these units of weight are called *Atomic Mass Units*). The half-lives of the three primordial radionuclides noted above are all very long and are measured in billions of years. Thus the amount of these particular radionuclides has not decayed to negligible levels over the past five billion or so years since the creation of the earth.

A third type of radionuclide is called man-made or *anthropogenic*. Although many of these radionuclides, including examples such as strontium-90 and plutonium-239, are formed by natural processes on the earth, their natural concentrations are so low as to be virtually undetectable. Most of the strontium-90 and plutonium-239 which can now be detected on the earth's surface comes from man-made sources, notably fallout from the above ground testing of nuclear weapons in the 1950s and early 1960s. Weapons testing also increased the

| RADIOACTIVE ATOMS AND THEIR HALF-LIVES | | |
|---|---|---|
| **Atom** | **Half-Life** | **Emitted Radiation\*** |
| Hydrogen-3 | 12.4 years | beta |
| Carbon-14 | 5,730 years | beta |
| Potassium-40 | 1.3 billion years | beta, gamma, x |
| Cobalt-60 | 5.3 years | beta, gamma |
| Strontium-90 | 29.1 years | beta |
| Iodine-131 | 8 days | beta, gamma, x |
| Thorium-232 | 14 billion years | alpha, gamma, x |
| Uranium-235 | 0.7 billion years | alpha, gamma, x |
| Uranium-238 | 4.5 billion years | alpha, beta, gamma, x, neutrons |
| Plutonium-239 | 24,100 years | alpha, gamma, x |

\* see page 9 for a description of emitted radiation

concentration of tritiated water (water in which some of the stable hydrogen has been replaced by tritium) in our immediate environment to about 100 times its natural level by 1963; since that time, the normal radioactive decay of tritium and the dilution of tritiated water from the atmosphere into the deep oceans are gradually returning the concentration of tritium in fresh water to its natural level. Tritium is also produced in nuclear power reactors, but very little of this tritium escapes into the environment. The various sources of radiation, man-made and natural, are described in more detail in Chapter 3.

Some radionuclides, for example tritium (hydrogen-3), carbon-14 and potassium-40, decay in a single step to a stable element. Other radionuclides, such as thorium-232 and uranium-238, form another radioactive atom during the first step in their normal decay. The offspring, or *decay products*, of thorium-232 go through a total of nine radioactive decays before reaching a stable atom, while the decay products of uranium-238 go through thirteen radioactive transformations before reaching a stable atom. Many heavier radionuclides, like thorium-232 and uranium-238, thus form the head of a decay series consisting of a sequence of radionuclides, each with its own characteristic half-life (Figure 2.3).

Uranium-238 is unusual in that it may on rare occasions also undergo a spontaneous *fission* into two smaller radioactive atoms with the liberation of neutrons (this is discussed more fully in Chapter 10).

FIGURE 2.3
RADIOACTIVE DECAY CHAIN

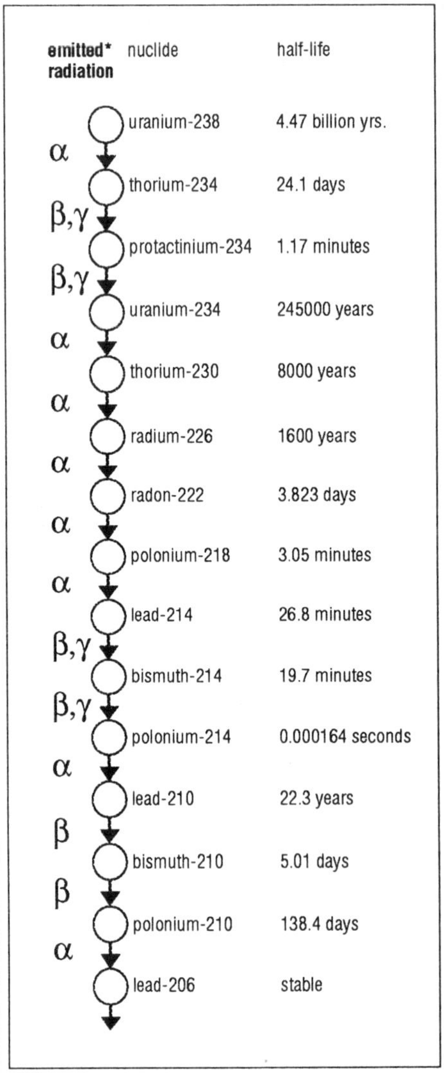

| emitted* radiation | nuclide | half-life |
|---|---|---|
| | uranium-238 | 4.47 billion yrs. |
| α | thorium-234 | 24.1 days |
| β,γ | protactinium-234 | 1.17 minutes |
| β,γ | uranium-234 | 245000 years |
| α | thorium-230 | 8000 years |
| α | radium-226 | 1600 years |
| α | radon-222 | 3.823 days |
| α | polonium-218 | 3.05 minutes |
| α | lead-214 | 26.8 minutes |
| β,γ | bismuth-214 | 19.7 minutes |
| β,γ | polonium-214 | 0.000164 seconds |
| α | lead-210 | 22.3 years |
| β | bismuth-210 | 5.01 days |
| β | polonium-210 | 138.4 days |
| α | lead-206 | stable |

* See page 9 for a description of the emitted radiation and Chapter 15 for symbols.

The strength or activity of a radioactive source is measured in *becquerel* (Bq). A source with an activity or strength of 1 Bq has one radioactive atom disintegrating every second. The concentration of radioactivity in gas, liquid, or a solid is commonly expressed as Bq per cubic metre, Bq per litre, and Bq per kilogram respectively. For example the concentration of radon-222 in air is typically about 30 Bq/m³, of radium-226 in municipal drinking water about 0.0003 Bq/litre and of potassium-40 in soil about 400 Bq/kg.

## WHAT IS IONIZING RADIATION?

Ionizing radiations are characterized by their ability to dissociate neutral atoms or combinations of atoms (*molecules*) in a gas into positively and negatively charged particles called *ions*. Ionization is discussed more fully later in this chapter. It was this property which was used in 1925 to devise the first practical method of measuring the strength of an ionizing radiation field.

X-rays, the first type of ionizing radiation to be discovered, are normally produced by accelerating a beam of electrons through a high voltage electrical field (usually about 150 thousand volts) in a vacuum. When these high speed electrons strike a solid target, for example, a plate made of tungsten, x-rays are emitted from the target (Figure 2.4).

| • Nucleus of Atom | Protons & Neutrons | Positive Charge |
|---|---|---|
| • Atom | Nucleus & orbital electrons | No net charge |
| • Molecule | Combinations of atoms with no unpaired orbital electrons | No net charge |
| • Ion | Electron, atom or molecule which has lost or gained one or more electrons | Positive or negative charge |

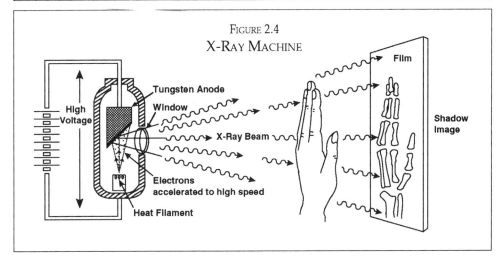

FIGURE 2.4
X-RAY MACHINE

X-rays from the sun, other stars and from the decay of certain radionuclides on earth can also be detected, by use of special instruments for this purpose, but the intensity of these sources of x-rays is extremely low at the surface of the earth. X-rays are part of the electromagnetic spectrum. Because x-rays have high energy compared to other forms of electromagnetic radiation, they can knock electrons from the atoms of the material through which they are passing. Both the electron produced and the atom left are ions and are electrically charged. Less energetic types of electromagnetic radiations such as visible light are not capable of disrupting or breaking up atoms in this way. In most of this document, when the term *radiation* is used it represents ionizing radiation.

Any subatomic particle moving at high speed is also included in the general category of ionizing radiation. The first three types of ionizing radiation from natural sources to be discovered were called *alpha, beta* and *gamma* rays, depending on the way in which their paths were bent in a strong magnetic field (Figure 2.5). The path of the alpha rays, now generally called alpha particles, was bent slightly to one side, showing that they carried a positive electrical charge and were fairly heavy, while beta rays or particles were bent strongly in the opposite direction, indicating that they carried a negative charge and were much lighter. Alpha rays are now known to be positively charged helium nuclei (two protons in combination with two neutrons)

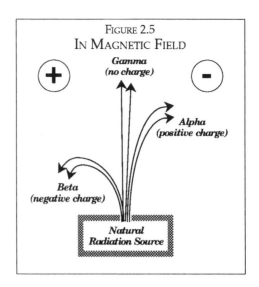

FIGURE 2.5
IN MAGNETIC FIELD

which are ejected from the heavy nuclei of radionuclides such as thorium-232 and uranium-238 in some of the steps in their natural decay processes. Beta rays or beta particles are high-speed, negatively charged electrons which are ejected from the nuclei of tritium and many other radionuclides. Radioactive decay usually results in the liberation of appreciable amounts of energy from the nucleus. This energy frequently appears as gamma rays. Gamma rays belong to the electromagnetic spectrum and are similar to x-rays. Their path does not bend in a magnetic field.

A variety of other subatomic particles have now been discovered. These include the *positron* which is a beta particle with a positive instead of a negative charge, and the *neutrino* which has zero charge. These particles are not of major concern in radiation protection.

For most practical purposes, the only other subatomic particle that is important in radiation protection is the neutron. Free neutrons outside the nucleus do occur at low levels in nature and are responsible for part of the cosmic radiation which reaches the earth's surface from outer space. Intense fields of neutrons are produced in nuclear reactors. Materials when bombarded by neutrons usually become radioactive but this does not normally occur when materials are bombarded by other common types of radiation such as gamma rays.

## INTERACTION OF IONIZING RADIATIONS WITH TISSUE

To understand the interaction of ionizing radiation with tissue it is necessary to understand a little about the molecular structure of materials.

Matter is made up from basic building blocks, either atoms or combinations of atoms, called molecules. The combinations result from the interaction of the orbital electrons of atoms. A simple example is a molecule of water which is a combination of one atom of oxygen with two atoms of hydrogen (Figure 2.6).

A variety of processes can *ionize* atoms and molecules. *Ionization* is the removal of an orbital electron from an atom or molecule, to create an *ion pair*. An ion pair consists of the removed electron (which may quickly attach itself to an other atom

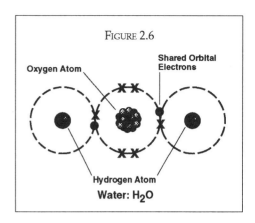

FIGURE 2.6

Oxygen Atom

Shared Orbital Electrons

Hydrogen Atom

**Water: $H_2O$**

to form a negative ion) and the residual atom, or molecule, which now has a positive charge. Producing ion pairs is the principal way in which energy is transferred from ionizing radiation to material, such as tissue, through which it is passing. The material or tissue is said to have received a radiation *dose*, which in its simplest form is measured by the energy absorbed, in joules per kilogram of tissue irradiated; (units of radiation dose more useful in radiation protection are discussed in detail later in this section). Alpha particles and to a lesser extent neutrons produce dense tracks of ionized particles as they pass through materials. The tracks of beta and gamma radiation have much less ionization per length of track (Figure 2.7).

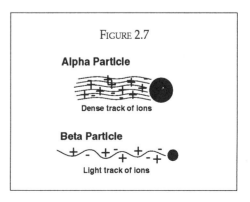

FIGURE 2.7

**Alpha Particle**

Dense track of Ions

**Beta Particle**

Light track of Ions

In the process of the deposition of energy in tissue (or other material) some very reactive chemicals, known as free radicals, are produced. These can cause potentially harmful chemical changes in the organic materials in the cells of the tissue.

```
┌─────────────────────────────────────┐
│   IONIZING RADIATION IN TISSUE       │
├─────────────────────────────────────┤
│              Radiation               │
│                 ⬇                    │
│     Energy deposition in tissue      │
│                 ⬇                    │
│     Reactive free radicals formed    │
│                 ⬇                    │
│          Chemical changes            │
│                 ⬇                    │
│          Biological effects          │
└─────────────────────────────────────┘
```

The organic molecule in tissue that is most important in the potential risk from ionizing radiation is *deoxyribonucleic acid* or *DNA*. The DNA molecule carries the blueprints for life; in humans, there are more than 10,000 instructions for life processes encoded along its length. Most of the chemical changes in the structure of DNA, whether these occur spontaneously or because of exposure to radiation or other agents, are actively repaired by living cells. The instructions for this repair are themselves encoded in the DNA. A small fraction of the DNA damage is not correctly repaired and thus results in permanent changes in the DNA structure. Some of these changes may find expression as a harmful biological effect, such as an inherited genetic defect or as a cancer. Alpha particles produce many sites of damage within a small distance of each other, so that errors in repair are more probable than for the changes caused by gamma rays, where the sites of damage are more widely scattered.

At radiation doses which are low enough to permit survival of the irradiated cell, the fraction of permanent changes with harmful biological effects is less than one in 10,000 of the total chemical changes produced in the DNA by the radiation.

An important characteristic of the various ionizing radiations is how deeply they can penetrate the body tissues. This depends on the energy of the radiation, its electrical charge and its mass. X-rays, gamma rays and neutrons of sufficient energy can reach all tissues of the body from an external source. Alpha particles, on the other hand, are stopped by a thin sheet of paper or by the superficial dead layers of the skin. Consequently, radionuclides which emit alpha particles are not hazardous to humans unless they are taken into the body. This may occur by inhalation (breathing in), ingestion (eating and drinking), or because of a wound becoming contaminated. The depth to which beta particles may penetrate body tissues depends upon their energy, which is in turn characteristic of the radionuclides from which they were derived. Energetic beta particles may penetrate a centimetre or so of tissue, although most are absorbed in the first few millimetres. Consequently, radionuclides which emit beta particles are hazardous to superficial tissues such as skin or the lenses of the eye, when these radionuclides are outside the body, but are only hazardous to internal tissues when taken into the body.

## Dose Quantities

Ionizing radiation cannot be directly detected by the human senses, but it can be detected and measured by a variety of physical methods. The methods of measurement have undergone many improvements, and the radiation dose units used have been modified several times since the ability to measure low doses of radiation was first established in 1925.

In radiation protection it is essential that the units used to measure radiation dose reflect the damage, or injury, that may result to tissue and organs from the dose received. There are three important factors associated with how much damage a given radiation exposure causes. The first is the amount of energy the radiation deposits in the tissue or organs of the body. This is known as the *absorbed dose*. The unit of absorbed dose is the *gray;* abbreviation Gy. One Gy is an absorbed dose of one joule per kilogram of material irradiated. A person who has received a whole body dose of 1 Gy has absorbed one joule of energy in each kilogram of body tissue.

Radiation damage to a specific organ or tissue of the body has been found to depend not only on the energy absorbed but also on the type of radiation that is depositing the energy. Absorbed dose is therefore multiplied by a *radiation weighting factor* to give an *equivalent dose* for the organ. X-rays, gamma rays and beta rays have been assigned a radiation weighting factor of one, and alpha particles and high speed neutrons, a factor of 20.

| RADIATION WEIGHTING FACTORS | |
|---|---|
| Type of Radiation | Factor |
| x, beta and gamma | 1 |
| Neutrons:   0.01 to 0.1 MeV* | 10 |
| 0.1 to 2 MeV | 20 |
| 2 to 20 MeV | 10 |
| Alpha particles | 20 |

*MeV is an abbreviation for million electron volts

The equivalent dose obtained by multiplying the absorbed dose by the radiation weighting factor is in units called *sieverts*, abbreviated as Sv. (Sievert and Gray are the names of distinguished scientists who made important contributions to radiation protection. The use of their names in this way parallels the use of the names of great scientists such as Watt, Joule and Newton.)

Sub-multiples of the sievert are in common use, such as the millisievert (mSv), which is one-thousandth of a sievert. The equivalent dose provides an index of the risk of harm from exposure of a specific organ or tissue to various types of ionizing radiation, whatever the type or energy: an equivalent dose of 1 Sv to the lung from alpha radiation for example, will cause the same harm as 1 Sv to the lung from x-rays.

However the harm induced by exposure to radiation varies appreciably, in both magnitude and kind from one tissue or organ of the body to another, for the same equivalent dose. The risk of fatal cancer resulting from an equivalent dose of 1 Sv to the lungs is greater than the risk of fatal cancer from an equivalent dose of 1 Sv to the thyroid, and the nature of the harm resulting from an equivalent dose of 1 Sv to the reproductive organs differs from the harm resulting from the same dose to the red bone marrow. To allow for this difference in harmful effects for the same equivalent dose, a set of *tissue weighting factors* has been developed. These tissue weighting factors are based on assessments of the probability of harm and the nature of the harm resulting from a given equivalent dose to the tissue. Factors which are included in the assessment are the probability of the induction of cancer, the relative ease with which the cancer can be cured, the probability that irradiation of the reproductive organs can result in serious genetic disorders in the offspring of irradiated persons, and the years of normal life expectancy lost or seriously impaired due to all these effects. The tissue weighting factors adopted by the International Commission on Radiological Protection in its 1990 recommendations are listed in the accompanying table.

When the absorbed doses in various tissues that have been irradiated are multiplied by both the radiation weighting factor and the tissue weighting factor and then summed, the result is called the *effective dose*. The unit of effective dose is also the sievert (Sv). For low levels of radiation the harm resulting from a given effective dose should be about the same regardless of the type of radiation or the tissues irradiated. Thus the amount of serious biological harm resulting from an effective dose of 1 Sv of alpha radiation to the lung should be roughly the same as

### TISSUE WEIGHTING FACTORS

| Tissue of Organ | Factor |
|---|---|
| Reproductive Organs | 0.20 |
| Red bone marrow | 0.12 |
| Colon | 0.12 |
| Lung | 0.12 |
| Stomach | 0.12 |
| Bladder | 0.05 |
| Breast | 0.05 |
| Liver | 0.05 |
| Oesophagus | 0.05 |
| Thyroid | 0.05 |
| Skin | 0.01 |
| Bone surface | 0.01 |
| Remainder | 0.05 |
| Whole body total | 1.0 |

that from an effective dose of 1 Sv of x-rays to the reproductive organs, or from 1 Sv of uniform whole body irradiation from high energy gamma rays.

As an example, if a man receives a whole body dose of 100 mSv and in addition an equivalent dose of 500 mSv to his thyroid and an equivalent dose of 400 mSv to his lungs, then his effective dose E is given by:

$$E = 1 \times \text{Whole Body Dose} + 0.05 \times \text{Thyroid Dose} + 0.12 \times \text{Lung Dose}$$
$$= 1 \times 100 + 0.05 \times 500 + 0.12 \times 400$$
$$= 100 + 25 + 48$$
$$= 173 \text{ mSv}$$

It is often useful to have a measure of the total radiation dose to a group of people or a whole population. The quantity used to express this total is the *collective dose.* The unit of collective dose is the *person sievert* (person·Sv). Collective dose is simply the sum of the effective doses received by each person in an exposed group of people. For example, if in a group of 100 workers, 20 each received 1 mSv dose, 30 each received 2 mSv dose and 50 each received 3 mSv dose, then the collective dose for this group is given by: Collective Dose = (20 x 1 + 30 x 2 + 50 x 3) = 230 person·mSv. Similarly, if we assume that the average individual dose from natural sources in Canada is about 2 mSv per year and that the population is about 27 million people, then the collective dose from natural sources of radiation is the product of these two numbers or about 54,000 person·Sv per year.

Another useful dose quantity is *committed dose.* Radionuclides with a long physical half-life, which are taken into the body, may remain in certain tissues for many days or years. The committed dose is the total effective dose received from a radioactive substance in the body, during 50 years after intake by a radiation worker or other adult, or during 70 years after intake by a child. This value varies greatly depending upon the internal metabolism and rate of elimination from the body of each individual radionuclide. Committed doses are implicitly included in any calculations of effective dose. Knowledge of effective dose units and collective dose units is sufficient to understand natural and man-made sources of radiation and their biological effects. Unless otherwise specified, use of the word *dose* in this document should be interpreted as being effective dose.

---

**HIERARCHY OF DOSE QUANTITIES**

Absorbed dose
(radiation energy deposited in a unit mass of tissue)

Equivalent dose
(absorbed dose weighted for harmfulness of different types of radiation)

Effective dose
(equivalent dose weighted for susceptibility of different tissues to radiation induced cancers or genetic disorders)

Collective dose
(effective doses to individuals summed over all exposed persons in the population)

---

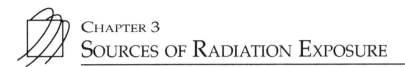

CHAPTER 3

# SOURCES OF RADIATION EXPOSURE

## EXPOSURE OF THE PUBLIC

Most of the radiation exposure of the public comes from natural sources. In Canada the total average dose from natural sources is about 2 mSv per year. Of this total, roughly one-third of a mSv per year comes from each of the following three sources: cosmic radiation from space, terrestrial gamma rays from the soil beneath our feet, and radiation from natural radionuclides, such as potassium-40, which are incorporated into our body. The rest comes from the inhalation of radon gases and their short-lived radioactive decay products in the air. Radon gases, which are chemically inert, are formed in the decay series from naturally occuring uranium and thorium. The majority of the exposure from this source is due to the short-lived decay products in the radioactive chain that starts with radon-222 in the uranium chain and ends with, but does not include, lead-210. Radon diffuses continuously out of the soil everywhere and accumulates in air inside houses. The dose resulting from inhalation of radon decay products in air is somewhat uncertain, as will be discussed in Chapter 4.

### AVERAGE ANNUAL EXPOSURE OF GENERAL PUBLIC IN CANADA TO IONIZING RADIATION

| Source | Dose mSv per yr |
|---|---|
| NATURAL | |
| Cosmic rays | 0.3 |
| Gamma rays from earth | 0.35 |
| Internal sources | 0.35 |
| Inhalation of radon decay products | 1.0 |
| Total (rounded) | 2.0 |
| MAN-MADE | |
| Medical diagnoses | 0.6 |
| Fallout from weapons testing | < 0.01 |
| Fallout from Chernobyl | < 0.001 |
| Nuclear power stations | < 0.001 |
| Other miscellaneous sources | 0.02 |
| Total (rounded) | 0.6 |

The largest man-made source of radiation exposure of the public is the use of medical x-rays for diagnostic purposes. The resulting doses vary considerably from one person to another. Reliable estimates of average doses from medical x-rays in Canada are not available. Based on some Canadian data and more detailed studies from the U.S.A. and the U.K., on average the total dose from medical x-rays plus other applications of ionizing radiation in medical diagnoses is currently estimated to be about 0.6 mSv per year.

Other sources of radiation arising from human activity add very little to this total. Annual doses from fallout from nuclear weapons testing reached a maximum in the 1950s and early 1960s but are currently so low as to be considered negligible in comparison with doses from natural sources. Doses from the catastrophic accident at Chernobyl in 1986 reached a maximum of about 0.002 mSv in Canada during the first year after the accident but are now insignificant. Doses received by members of the public from nuclear power generating stations in Canada are also low. Maximum doses for individuals living near a nuclear power station are estimated to be less than 0.05 mSv per year, while doses for persons who live further away from these stations are smaller still. The average dose for persons living in Ontario from the nuclear power stations, that currently supply about half the province's electricity, is less than 0.001 mSv per year and the average exposure from nuclear power stations to all persons in Canada is even smaller.

There are a number of other human activities that increase our exposure to radiation by a small amount. A flight of 10 hours in a commercial jet aircraft at an average altitude of eight kilometres will result in an increased dose from cosmic radiation of about 0.02 mSv; the average dose to all Canadians from this source is about 0.005 mSv per year. Other sources of increased radiation exposure include the use of phosphate fertilizers, various mining activities, the use of coal for production of electricity, and pumping water from deep wells (it contains radon). Total average exposures of individuals in the public from all these miscellaneous sources are probably in the region of 0.02 mSv per year.

All of the exposures given above represent average values. There are considerable variations in radiation doses from natural sources from one location to another in Canada. Living at higher altitudes results in an increase in exposure to cosmic rays. Populations living in cities such as Bogota, Lhasa, or Quito, which are all at an altitude of three kilometres or more, receive about 1 mSv per year from cosmic radiation, but there are no major cities in Canada at these altitudes. The doses from cosmic radiation in cities at about one kilometre altitude in western Canada are only about 0.4 mSv per year as compared to the average value of 0.3 mSv per year for all of Canada. These variations due to altitude are much smaller than the variations in gamma ray exposures from the ground which may vary tenfold or more at different locations in Canada (see Figure 3.1). The values shown in this figure are those measured outdoors. Gamma exposures may be slightly lower indoors in houses of wooden frame construction, and slightly higher in concrete basements or in masonry houses.

There is no practical method of reducing natural exposures from cosmic rays, gamma rays from the earth or internal radionuclides such as potassium-40. In contrast, it is fairly easy to reduce the high concentrations of radon decay

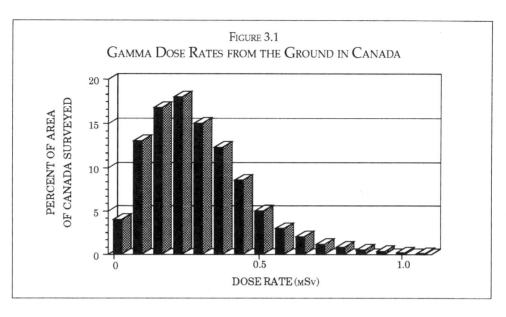

FIGURE 3.1
GAMMA DOSE RATES FROM THE GROUND IN CANADA

PERCENT OF AREA OF CANADA SURVEYED

DOSE RATE (MSV)

products which may occur in the air in some existing homes and to minimize these concentrations when building new homes. The average concentration in houses in different cities in Canada varies by about tenfold, depending on the type of soil found in the local area. The variation in radon decay product concentrations in air in individual homes across Canada may be a thousand-fold or more.

### APPROXIMATE AVERAGE EXPOSURES TO RADON DECAY PRODUCTS IN THE AIR OF HOUSES IN SEVEN CANADIAN CITIES

| City | mSv per year |
|---|---|
| Vancouver | 0.2 |
| Montreal | 0.4 |
| Toronto | 0.55 |
| Edmonton | 0.8 |
| Halifax | 1.2 |
| Regina | 1.6 |
| Winnipeg | 2.2 |
| Population average for Canada | about 0.8 |

## OCCUPATIONAL EXPOSURES

Occupational exposures are discussed in detail in Chapter 10. Doses received by individual workers are on average quite low but may occasionally approach the current annual limit of 50 mSv and on rare occasions exceed that value. In 1990 there were about 111,000 radiation workers in Canada and the average dose they received in that year was about 0.5 mSv, which is a population dose of 55.5 person·Sv. If this is averaged over the entire Canadian population then, occupational exposures contributed about 0.002 mSv to the average radiation dose of 2.6 mSv in Canada.

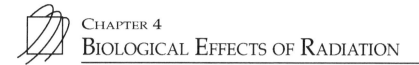

# CHAPTER 4
# BIOLOGICAL EFFECTS OF RADIATION

## EARLY EFFECTS OF HIGH DOSES

High doses of radiation delivered at high dose rates, for example 5 Sv in a few minutes, can produce a variety of effects in humans, including death, within a few months. High doses, in a short time, kill so many cells in certain tissues that the body cannot cope with this damage. These early effects are characterized by the existence of a *threshold dose* below which the effects are not observed. Doses below 1 Sv in a few minutes do not result in any early deaths. Internationally accepted dose limits are intended to prevent the occurrence of any of these early effects. The internationally recommended dose limit for workers in the unlikely event of a nuclear emergency is 0.5 Sv to the whole body (or 5 Sv from beta rays to the skin) in a short period. The ability of high radiation doses delivered at high dose rates to kill living cells has been well known for many years and was successfully used to cure a skin cancer in 1899. This property of high radiation doses is still applied in cancer treatment.

| DOSE (Sv) | EFFECT |
|---|---|
| 0 - 0.25 | No obvious injury |
| 0.25-1 | Temporary nausea, temporary sterility in males and temporary blood cell changes are all possible; no early deaths. |
| 1 - 3 | Nausea, fatigue and vomiting, blood cell changes, loss of appetite, diarrhoea; temporary sterility in males; death possible. |
| 3 - 6 | Nausea and vomiting, diarrhoea, marked blood cell changes, loss of weight, general malaise; early death of 50 % of those exposed; permanent sterility and eye cataract development in survivors. |

## LATE EFFECTS OF LOW DOSES

Although low doses of radiation do not produce any early effects, they may result in late effects which do not become evident until many years after exposure. Late effects of primary concern are an increased incidence of cancer in exposed persons, and of genetic disorders in their children. These late effects are due to damage to DNA, as noted in Chapter 2.

---

Data on radiation-induced cancers are derived from the follow-up of groups of persons who were exposed to relatively high doses of radiation many years ago. These groups of persons include early radium dial painters who inadvertently swallowed appreciable amounts of radium during their work; patients treated with high doses of medical x-rays to cure a crippling arthritic disease of the backbone; uranium miners who inhaled high concentrations of radon decay products in mine air at a time when the hazards of this source of radiation were not fully appreciated; and the Japanese bomb survivors who were exposed to high doses of gamma radiation to the whole body in August 1945.

The types of cancer caused by radiation are the same as those that occur naturally. However the risk of an increased incidence of cancers per unit of radiation dose can be estimated by careful follow-up of groups of persons who were exposed in the past to high doses of radiation.

Not all cancers are fatal. About 95% of all lung cancers, about 50% of breast cancers, 10% of thyroid cancers and 0.2% of all skin cancers are fatal. One third of cancers of internal organs caused by radiation are thought to be curable. If skin cancers are included, then the percentage of cancers that can be cured is much higher. However, the risk of fatal cancers is the principal concern in radiation protection. Estimation of fatal cancer risks also helps in comparing the risks of radiation with other fatal risks encountered in life. The comparisons of nonfatal risks are fraught with difficulty.

The risk of radiation-induced genetic disorders cannot be determined by direct study of human populations. Despite extensive efforts, no significant increase in genetic disorders has been detected in the children of the Japanese bomb survivors at Hiroshima and Nagasaki, and there is no other reliable evidence to contradict this finding.

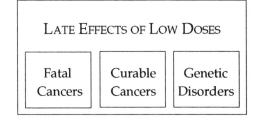

QUANTITATIVE ASSESSMENT OF CANCER RISKS

Estimates of the probability that a given dose of radiation will result in the appearance of cancer in exposed persons are provided by international scientific committees which are appointed for that purpose. The *United Nations Scientific Committee on the Effects of Atomic Radiation* (UNSCEAR) was established in 1955 because of concern about the potential health effects of radioactive fallout. This committee currently meets once a year in Vienna and consists of 70-100 scientists (physicists, biologists, geneticists, medical doctors and others) from more than 20 countries. A senior representative from Health Canada is currently head of the Canadian delegation, with scientific advisors appointed from the Atomic Energy Control Board and other agencies. At about five-year intervals UNSCEAR produces a voluminous document reviewing recent scientific publications on the levels of radiation to which humans are exposed and the biological effects of ionizing radiation.

The *International Commission on Radiological Protection*, or ICRP, was formed (under a different name) in 1928 and dealt initially with protection against undue exposure to medical x-rays and to radium. With the advent of nuclear weapons, nuclear reactors and high energy accelerators, this committee was reorganized and given its present name in 1950.

Thirteen scientists who are selected for their expertise comprise the main commission; they come from such countries as Argentina, China, England, France, Germany, Italy, Japan, Poland, Russia and the U.S.A. In addition, the ICRP has four permanent committees composed of scientists with expertise in different radiation protection specialties. It also establishes working groups to deal with selected topics and can call upon experts from laboratories around the world. The ICRP reviews the scientific literature on biological effects of radiation and issues reports with recommendations on various aspects of the protection of humans against all sources of ionizing radiation. A third important source of information on potential health effects of radiation are the reports of the U.S. committees on the *Biological Effects of Ionizing Radiation* (BEIR). These committees operate under the auspices of the U.S. National Academy of Sciences and are funded by the Environmental Protection Agency. The most recent report was produced by 12 representatives from universities and hospitals in North America plus five representatives from various national laboratories in the U.S.A. The reports of this U.S. Committee are completely independent of those produced by UNSCEAR and frequently adopt a different approach to analysis of the data on the health effects of radiation. Like UNSCEAR, the BEIR reports are concerned only with the assessment of effects and do not make any recommendations on radiation protection.

Each industrialized country also has its own national committee on radiation protection. In Canada, this role is filled by the *Advisory Committee on Radiological Protection* (ACRP), which reports directly to the president of the Canadian regulatory agency, the Atomic Energy Control Board. The ACRP reviews published literature on health effects of radiation, co-sponsors public scientific symposia on relevant topics, and makes recommendations on dose limits in Canada. This Committee currently consists of medical persons, plus others from across Canada selected for their expertise in different scientific areas. The recommendations of the national committees in Canada and in other countries closely follow the recommendations of the ICRP.

## Flow of Information

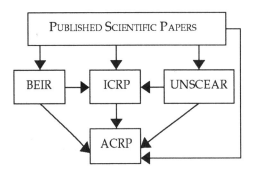

The most recent assessments, by all four of the above committees, of the total fatal cancers produced by whole body irradiation are based on the Japanese bomb survivor data. The registered bomb survivors for whom dose estimates are available are a group of about 42,000 persons of all ages and both sexes who were exposed in 1945 to a wide range of doses in a short time. In addition there is a control group of nearly equal size, who were too far away from the centre of the bomb explosions to receive any appreciable radiation dose from this source. Follow-up of these persons from 1950 to 1985 has produced sufficient data to be statistically reliable. Dose estimation for the survivors has not been simple and is reviewed occasionally. An international effort to reassess the radiation doses received by each of the bomb survivors resulted in improved estimates in 1986. The characteristics of this group of persons are summarized in the accompanying table.

### Follow-Up of Registered Bomb Survivors 1950 –1985

| Group | Number |
|---|---|
| Exposed group of persons | 41,719 |
| Control, non-exposed group | 34,272 |
| Total persons in both groups | 75,991 |
| Total deaths in both groups 1950 – 1985 | 28,737 |
| Total cancer deaths in exposed group | 3,435 |
| Cancer deaths in exposed group attributable to radiation exposure in 1945 | 340 |

Over 60% of the registered bomb survivors were still alive at the end of 1985. The exposed group received varying doses in 1945 ranging from 10 mSv to about 5,000 mSv. In this group about 10% of all cancer deaths up to 1985, or about 2% of all deaths in the group, are currently attributed to their radiation exposures. There has not been any increase in deaths due to causes other than cancer in the bomb survivors who received radiation doses less than 2000 mSv in 1945; these results substantiate independent data obtained in studies on animals.

Many problems must be considered in order to use the observed data on excess cancers in Japanese bomb survivors to make an assessment of the lifetime probability of radiation-induced cancer at *lower* doses of radiation at *lower* dose rates.

The first problem is how to use (extrapolate) the data on the increased numbers of cancers experienced by the Japanese survivors in the first 40 years after exposure to predict the increase that will occur over the total lifespan of the population. Various models which relate the increase of cancer with age after exposure have been used to obtain this lifetime risk value.

A second problem is how to apply the lifetime risk of various cancers occurring in a Japanese population to other countries in which the normal patterns of cancer incidence are different. The 1991 ICRP estimates, which are intended to provide values representative of an international population, were the average results obtained using two different extrapolation models and applying them to the population of five countries.

---

PROBLEMS IN ESTIMATING
CANCER RISKS FROM WHOLE
BODY IRRADIATION

- Extrapolation from limited data to lifetime cancer risks.

- Extrapolation from Japanese data to other countries.

- Extrapolation from observed effects at high dose rate to expected effects at low dose rate.

- Impossibility of proving a linear relationship down to low doses.

---

A third problem is the extrapolation from observed data on excess cancers in the Japanese bomb survivors, who were exposed to various whole body doses of gamma radiation in about a second, to predicted effects of radiation at low dose rate. The 1991 recommendations of the ICRP, which had both the 1988 UNSCEAR and 1990 BEIR reports available for consideration, chose to use a dose-rate effectiveness factor of two; that is, a radiation dose delivered at low dose rate is about half as effective in producing long-term harmful effects as the same dose delivered at high dose rate.

A final problem is the applicability of the data to persons exposed to very low radiation doses. The ICRP and other scientific committees have assumed for many years that *any* increase in radiation exposure will result in a proportional increase in radiation-induced cancers. This assumption is impossible to prove; even for the Japanese bomb survivors, there was no significant excess of cancers at radiation doses below 200 mSv, although the data are compatible with a linear relationship between dose and effect at all doses. In Canada, the ACRP has considered this linear relationship between dose and effect a reasonable and prudent assumption but, noting the difficulties involved in proving it, has recommended that we should speak of the *potential* increase in fatal cancers caused by low radiation exposures.

Despite these problems and the uncertainties involved in the various extrapolations noted above, a best estimate of the probability of radiation-induced cancers is needed for use in radiation protection. In 1991, the ICRP recommended the use of a value of four fatal cancers per 100 person·Sv for workers and five fatal cancers per 100 person·Sv for a general population of all ages. This would mean that the collective dose of about 50,000 person·Sv per year from natural sources of radiation in Canada could potentially account for 2,500 fatal cancers per year. This is a small fraction of the total number of fatal cancers which occur normally in Canada.

| HARM PER 100 PERSON.SV OF EXPOSURE | |
| --- | --- |
| WORKERS (AGE 18-65) | |
| Fatal Cancers | 4 |
| Total Harm* | 5.6 |
| GENERAL PUBLIC (ALL AGES) | |
| Fatal Cancers | 5 |
| Total Harm* | 7.3 |

\* Includes fatal and non-fatal cancers and serious genetic effects.

In addition to risks for radiation-induced cancer, there are nominal risk values for total harm produced by all the late effects of exposure to low doses of radiation. The values include four components: fatal cancers produced in different tissues; non-fatal or curable cancers produced in the same tissues; serious genetic disorders developing in offspring summed over all subsequent generations; and years of normal life expectancy lost or seriously impaired because of each of these late effects. When calculated as recommended by the ICRP, fatal cancers account for about 70% of the total harm. In Canada, the ACRP has recommended that these values for total harm should be adopted for use in radiation protection.

As noted earlier in Chapter 3, a considerable portion of our exposure to radiation from natural sources stems from inhalation of radon decay products in the air. The risk of lung cancer associated with breathing radon decay products is derived from follow-up of miners who were exposed in the past to high concentrations of these contaminants in mine air.

Four of the eight major published studies on this topic relate to mining sites in Canada. The available data on effects of exposure to radon decay products are normally expressed in terms of an old unit, the *Working Level Month*, or *WLM*, (see Glossary for WLM definition.) The ACRP in Canada has recently reviewed scientific publications on this topic and reconfirmed an earlier estimate that the lifetime risk of lung cancer following inhalation of radon decay products is about three per 10,000 miners exposed to one WLM each. The 1990 ICRP recommendations give a range from one to four fatal lung cancers per 10,000 miners per WLM. Most miners in the studies were cigarette smokers, and there are some problems in the extrapolation of these data to non-smokers and to children in the general population. There are also uncertainties in converting exposures in WLM into an effective dose in mSv. The ACRP has suggested that this conversion factor could be in the region of 5 mSv effective dose per WLM. This value was used to calculate the average exposures to radon from natural sources that were presented in Chapter 3.

## Quantitative Assessment of Genetic Risks

Assessment of genetic risks is carried out by the same scientific committees that are responsible for assessment of potential cancer risks. This assessment is more difficult than that for the risk of cancer because there has been no significant increase in disorders of genetic or partially genetic origin in any exposed populations studied. Therefore, other approaches to this topic have been devised. One approach is to measure the natural incidence of genetic disorders in the normal populations of various countries, to estimate the natural rate of spontaneous genetic mutations that are responsible for this natural incidence and then to measure the rates at which radiation produces genetic mutations in laboratory studies of mice and other animals. Canadian scientists have made important contributions to the first two items above; most of the work on mutation rates in irradiated mice has been carried out in the U.S.A. and the U.K..

---

### Data Needed to Estimate Genetic Risks

- Normal incidence of genetic disorders

- Natural rate of genetic mutations

- Rate of induced mutations per Sv

---

There are however some genetic disorders which occur naturally but are not produced by radiation. Certain disorders such as Down Syndrome are caused by an incorrect number of chromosomes in the fertilized egg cell, not by a mutation. This disorder, also known by the technical term "trisomy 21", occurs in about one of every 1,000 children born. Radiation geneticists who participated in preparation of recent BEIR and UNSCEAR reports agree that radiation is unlikely to cause Down Syndrome or other related disorders that are due to an incorrect number of chromosomes in the fertilized egg.

A well-established principle in genetics is that organisms with serious genetic mutations, whether produced spontaneously, by toxic chemicals, by viruses or by radiation, do not reproduce as well as organisms which lack them. Consequently, serious genetic disorders tend to die out within a few generations in natural populations. The same principle can be applied to serious genetic disorders in human populations, especially to those disorders which become apparent in childhood, even though major medical advances have been made in the treatment of some of them. The incidence of serious genetic disorders that are induced by exposure of parents to radiation or other agents should therefore be highest in the first generation of children of the exposed persons. This increased incidence should gradually decrease in each successive generation. National and international scientific committees which review the genetic data have produced estimates not only of the probability of serious genetic disorders in the immediate children of irradiated parents but also of the probability summed over all subsequent generations. These latter estimates are used in the 1990 ICRP recommendations in the assessment of the risk of serious genetic disorders after exposure of parents to radiation. This estimate is 2.5 per 100 person·Sv for radiation received by parents any time before reproduction.

| FREQUENCY OF SERIOUS GENETIC DISORDERS PER 100 PERSON·SV | |
| --- | --- |
| Prior to reproduction (age 0 to about 30) | 2.5 |
| Average for workers (age 18 to 65) | 0.6 |
| Average for general public (all ages) | 1.0 |

Irradiation of the germ cells in the reproductive organs (ovaries and testes) is potentially harmful only if it occurs before or during the reproductive period of life. For those who will not subsequently have children, there is, by definition, no genetic risk. The fraction of a group of people for whom irradiation of the reproductive organs has genetic significance depends on the ages of the people involved. Assuming an average age of child bearing of 30 years and a life expectancy of 75 years, then the average risk of serious genetic disease resulting from irradiation of the whole population would

be 30/75 or 40% of that following the irradiation of younger people before reproduction. The corrected average genetic risk coefficients for irradiation of the public and the radiation workers are shown in the accompanying table. Using the best risk data available, exposure of the reproductive organs to natural background radiation in Canada is estimated to contribute 0.3% of the normal incidence of serious genetic disorders in Canada.

The probabilities of genetic effects discussed above refer to those inherited disorders which appear in the children and all subsequent descendants of persons whose reproductive organs were exposed to radiation before their children were conceived. These genetic effects must be clearly distinguished from any late effects of direct irradiation of the developing child in the womb of a pregnant mother.

## EXPOSURE DURING PREGNANCY

The developing child in the womb is believed to be particularly susceptible to the effects of high doses of radiation. Concern about this problem led to restrictions on the employment of women of reproductive age as radiation workers as early as 1945 in Canada. As more scientific knowledge about the effects of radiation on the embryo in early pregnancy accumulated, these restrictions on employment of women were dropped by the regulatory agency in Canada in 1985 and by the ICRP in 1991. It is now known that any effects of low level radiation on the developing child should be very close to zero during the first four weeks after conception, that is, during the first six weeks after onset of the last maternal menses. After a female radiation worker has declared her pregnancy to her employer, special restrictions on radiation exposure of the pregnant woman are imposed.

Exposure of the developing child in the womb to high doses of radiation at high dose rates may produce a variety of serious health effects, including congenital abnormalities and severe mental retardation in live-born children. However, no detectable effects of this kind are produced by low radiation doses below 0.1 Sv.

A major concern in radiation protection is the induction of cancer in children after exposure to low doses of radiation in the womb. Small but measurable increases in the incidence of childhood cancer were observed in studies of large numbers of children in the U.K. and U.S.A. whose mothers had received, in the 1940s and 1950s, medical diagnostic x-rays of the abdomen during their pregnancy. There is also some scanty and incomplete evidence for the appearance of excess cancers in adult life after exposure of developing children in the womb to high radiation doses at Hiroshima and Nagasaki. The 1990 ICRP recommendations assumed that the total probability of fatal cancers appearing later in life

after exposure of the developing child in the womb "is, at most, a few times that for the population as a whole." Using a few reasonable assumptions which are consistent with the ICRP report, and making some allowances for potential genetic effects due to irradiation of the child's reproductive organs, it can be calculated that the total potential detriment per Sv following radiation exposure in the womb is probably three to five times greater than that predicted for exposure of the population as a whole. Much of this calculated detriment is due to induction of childhood cancers, which result in a large loss of life expectancy per fatal cancer.

| Effect | Natural Frequency per 10,000 Live Births | Additional Cases per 10,000 after Exposure to 10mSv in the Womb |
|---|---|---|
| Spontanueous Abortions | 3,000 - 5,000 per 10,000 conceptions | none |
| Congenital Anomalies Evident within 2 years after birth | 600 - 800 | none |
| Severe Mental Retardation | about 80 | none |
| Childhood Cancers | 20 | 5 |
| Lifetime Fatal Cancers | about 2,500 | 15 |
| Serious Genetic Defects | about 2,500 | 2 |

## LATENCY PERIOD FOR LATE EFFECTS

Leukaemia (except chronic lymphatic leukaemia) will start to appear in a population in excess of its normal incidence about two years after the population has received a single high radiation exposure; this two years is called the minimum latency period. The excess leukaemias reach a maximum about eight years after radiation exposure and gradually decrease again to approach zero by about 30 or 40 years after exposure.

The appearance of excess lung cancers in miners exposed to high concentrations of radon daughters appears to follow a similar pattern. The minimum latency period is about five years; the excess lung cancers reach a maximum after about 10 to 15 years and then gradually taper off again. The minimum latency period for solid cancers (cancers other than leukaemia), in the Hiroshima and Nagasaki bomb survivors is about 10 years. The total number of radiation-induced cancers of this type in this group up to 1985 was 3.3 times the total number of radiation-induced leukaemias.

The risk models used in the 1990 ICRP recommendations indicate that the largest number of radiation-induced cancers will appear late in life at age 70-80 when the normal incidence of cancers from other causes is at its highest. On the other hand, most of the childhood cancers which might be attributed to radiation exposure in the womb appear at age 3-5.

| AVERAGE AGE AT WHICH LATE EFFECTS OF RADIATION APPEAR | |
|---|---|
| Leukaemia: | 8 to 10 years after irradiation |
| Solid Cancers: | Age 70 |
| Childhood Cancers: | Age 3 – 5 |
| Genetic Effects: | Non-Detectable |

As noted earlier, the frequency of serious genetic disorders that are induced by radiation would be highest in the first generation of children of exposed parents and gradually decrease in subsequent generations. This theoretical prediction cannot be confirmed because the effects of radiation are so small that no significant excess of genetic disorders can be detected in humans, either in the children of the Japanese bomb survivors or in persons who have lived for many generations in areas of the world where exposures to radiation from natural sources are higher than average, such as parts of China.

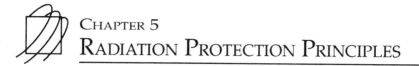

CHAPTER 5
# RADIATION PROTECTION PRINCIPLES

## BASIC PHILOSOPHY

Approaches to radiation protection are remarkably consistent throughout the world. This is due largely to the International Commission on Radiological Protection (ICRP). The ICRP is a non-governmental scientific organization which has published recommendations for protection against ionizing radiation for over half a century. Its authority derives from the scientific standing of its members and the merit of its recommendations. Governments in various countries, including Canada, evaluate the recommendations and put them into practice in a manner appropriate to their circumstances.

Radiation protection is concerned with the protection of individuals, their offspring, and humankind as a whole, while still allowing necessary activities from which radiation exposure might result. In 1977 the ICRP identified two principal aims in radiation protection. The first is to prevent any early effects resulting from high radiation doses. The second is to limit the probability of radiation-induced cancers and serious genetic disorders to levels deemed to be acceptable to society. The present system of radiation protec-

tion is based on three central requirements, which have been outlined by the ICRP and strongly endorsed by the Advisory Committee on Radiological Protection (ACRP) in Canada. Each of these requirements involves social considerations. There is therefore considerable need for careful judgement.

## CENTRAL REQUIREMENTS FOR RADIATION PROTECTION

### JUSTIFICATION OF A PRACTICE

No practice involving exposure to radiation should be adopted unless it produces sufficient benefit to offset any radiation detriment it may cause.

### OPTIMIZATION OF PROTECTION

All exposures should be kept as low as reasonably achievable (ALARA), economic and social factors being taken into account.

### INDIVIDUAL DOSE LIMITS

The exposure of individuals from all relevant practices should be subject to regulatory dose limits, in order to ensure that no individual is exposed to radiation risks that are judged to be unacceptable in any normal circumstances.

## JUSTIFICATION

Most national decisions about human activities in society are based on implicit balancing of costs and benefits. This balancing leads to the conclusion that a chosen practice is, or is not, worthwhile. This is the 'Justification' process. Radiation effects must be regarded as one cost of any proposal involving increased exposure to radiation. However, the questions involved in the general principle of justification extend beyond radiation protection and may be illustrated by the nuclear power program. One basic question is the health effects of nuclear power and other sources of energy. Various research centres in Canada and other countries have made a major resource commitment to estimating the risks to health attributable to the production of electricity from different sources. Health risks from all stages of the fuel cycle are included. These are:

- mining of uranium ore or coal and drilling for oil or natural gas,

- processing and transportation of the fuel,

- utilization of the fuel to produce electricity, and

- disposal of used fuel residues.

Total risks to health of both workers and the public are calculated per unit of electrical power produced. These assessments have concentrated on health effects which can be predicted to result within the next 50–100 years because of current operations. The Advisory Committee on Nuclear Safety in Canada has recently reviewed these studies. The conclusion from this and other reviews is that in the production of electricity, coal is the fuel most hazardous to health, followed in order by oil, nuclear and natural gas. Preliminary calculations have been carried out on health hazards associated with the production of electricity from renewable sources of energy. These indicate that renewable sources such as hydraulic, wind and solar heat are somewhat more hazardous than nuclear

| FATALITIES* FROM THE OPERATION FOR 1 YEAR OF A 1 GIGAWATT ELECTRICAL STATION | | | |
|---|---|---|---|
| Type of Station | Workers | Public | Total |
| Coal | 1.6 | 4.5 – 7 | 6.1 – 8.6 |
| Oil | 0.22 – 0.53 | 0.3 – 30 | 0.5 – 30 |
| Hydro | 0.33 – 0.9 | 0.005 – 0.012 | 0.33 – 0.91 |
| Nuclear | 0.2 – 0.23 | 0.02 – 0.12 | 0.22 – 0.35 |
| Natural Gas | 0.13 – 0.3 | 0.006 – 0.35 | 0.14 – 0.65 |

* Estimated by the Advisory Committee on Nuclear Safety or from References in their 1987 Report

power stations, when accidents that occur during the manufacture, construction, and maintenance of facilities to utilize renewable sources are taken into account. However it should be noted that the total differences are on average only in the region of 10 to 20 fold.

Regulatory and other government agencies in our society consider that use of these sources is justified, provided that exposures of humans to radiation, other toxic agents and injuries are kept at a low level. Strategic and economic factors also need to be considered, for instance the diversity, security, cost, availability and reserves of various fuels. The construction and operating costs of various types of power stations, the expected demand for electricity, the need for a back-up source of power, and the environmental impact must also be included in the choice of an energy source. Radiation effects are therefore only one element in the complicated process of making a final choice.

---

JUSTIFICATION FOR SOURCES OF ELECTRICITY

- Health benefits versus health detriment
- Relative Costs
- Fuel Supplies
- Environmental Impact

---

The regulation and control of many human activities affecting our health and well being is part of an ongoing international process. This process has increased life expectancy in industrialized countries by 30 to 40 years during the past century, and continues to increase our current average life expectancy. Since 1965 the average rate of increase in life expectancy in Canada is about 65 days per year. Despite our best efforts to conserve energy, the demand for electricity is likely to continue to increase worldwide. This demand is closely linked to industrial prosperity in different areas of the world. The beneficial effects of cheap and safe sources of energy on our life expectancy and prosperity are a major factor to be considered in the process of justification.

## OPTIMIZATION

Once a practice has been selected and justified, the conduct of the chosen practice should be adjusted to maximize the benefits to the individual and to society. The basis of the ICRP recommendation is that all radiation exposures should be kept **As Low As Reasonably Achievable**, economic and social factors being taken into account. This concept, known as the ALARA concept, has been firmly established in radiation protection for many years, and is currently being broadened to address other aspects of health protection.

The ICRP recommendations of 1954 include the statement that no increment in radiation dose can be regarded as absolutely safe. This reasonable but unprovable assumption has led to the use of phrases such as "deadly radiation" in the popular press, and among some members of the public has aroused fears of any increase in exposure to radiation or other man-made cancer-causing agent. These natural human fears are usually based on a lack of understanding about the impact of various human activities on our health. Some basic guidelines on optimization published by the ICRP in 1989 are relevant to this problem. The ICRP has said "It is not possible to reduce radiation exposures from man's practices to zero increment over background without totally foregoing the benefits from the practices giving rise to the exposure. As a general guide, the amount of resources devoted to reducing radiation exposure has to be compared with resources devoted to other needs of society. Overall the objective is optimum resource allocation for safety and protection. Good practice generally in relation to health and safety must surely have the same overall objective."

---

KEEPING DOSES LOW

- Design of good facilities
- Training of operating personnel
- Professional judgement and advice
- Cost-benefit analysis

---

Efforts to keep radiation doses as low as reasonably achievable have in the past relied on design of good facilities, training of operating personnel and the day-to-day use of professional judgement and common sense. These efforts have been remarkably successful.

Quantitative techniques such as cost-benefit analysis are being used increasingly in making judgements. This method requires a decision on the amount of money that should be spent to reduce radiation doses. Society has a limited amount of resources available to reduce the risks from exposure to radiation and the risks of disease or premature death from all other causes. An ultimate financial limit is imposed by the total value of the gross domestic product per person in society. Researchers studying this topic have suggested that expenditures in the region of 50,000 to 200,000 dollars might be appropriate for society to spend to save a life or prevent serious injury. Any expenditures which are greatly in excess of these values are not of real benefit to society. They result in a waste of lives which could have been saved in other areas. The financial costs for improvements in radiation protection must be considered against other ways of spending money on safety. It can be argued, for example, that greater gains may be achieved by directing the funds to improved medical care or highway safety, or to reducing the non-radiation hazards in a nuclear facility.

The requirement to keep radiation exposures as low as reasonably achievable, economic and social factors being taken into account, is an overriding concern in radiation protection. Emphasis on this principle has kept average exposures of workers and of the public from man-made sources down to very low levels.

## INDIVIDUAL DOSE LIMITS

The ICRP has recommended that individual dose limits must also be applied. This is to be certain that no individual in society is exposed to an unacceptable degree of risk because of activities involving increased exposure to radiation. Considerable attention has been devoted to the topic of acceptable risks in society.

Canadian regulatory dose limits have been based on the recommendations that have been made by the ICRP since the 1950s. Dose limits recently proposed by the federal government follow the latest (1990) recommendations of the ICRP.

### CURRENT AND PROPOSED DOSE LIMITS* IN CANADA (mSv)

| Population Group | Current Limits | | Proposed Limit | |
|---|---|---|---|---|
| | Annual | Quarter Year | Over 5 Years | Annual |
| Workers | 50 | 30 | 100 | 50 |
| Public | 5 | - | - | 1 |

* Other limits exist for specific organs and tissues

A risk-free society is unobtainable. There is risk in all human activities (or lack of activity) although many risks are quite low. We appear to be willing to accept risk so as to enjoy the benefits of modern society, if the risks are not excessive or easily avoided. Studies of human psychology have indicated that a continuing annual chance of death of one in 100 due to fatal hazards at work would be clearly unacceptable in modern society. But an annual probability of dying of one in 1,000 due to hazards at work might be acceptable if the individual worker knew of the situation, judged that he or she had some offsetting benefit, and understood that everything reasonable had been done to reduce the risk.

The radiation dose limits recommended by the ICRP in 1977 and in 1990 were based on the assumption that an annual probability of death of one in 1,000 due to radiation exposure at work would be at the border of being unacceptable. There are of course occupations in Canada, notably commercial fishing and hunting, where occupational risks of fatal accidents exceed one in 1,000 per year.

Most radiation-induced fatal cancers occur late in life, while the average age of persons killed in conventional accidents at work is less than 40 years. The resultant loss of life expectancy from conventional occupational accidents is greater than for radiation induced fatalities. For continuing exposure to a given level of risk from age 18 to age 65, the average loss of life expectancy from a fatal accident is

| AVERAGE ANNUAL RISK OF DEATH IN CANADA FROM FATAL ACCIDENTS AT WORK AND FROM RADIATION EXPOSURE | |
|---|---|
| **Occupation** | **Risk of Death per Year** |
| Finance | 1 in 60,000 |
| Service | 1 in 40,000 |
| Trade | 1 in 20,000 |
| 2 mSv radiation per year | 1 in 12,000 |
| Government (includes police and firefighters) | 1 in 11,000 |
| Manufacturing | 1 in 11,000 |
| Transportation | 1 in 4,000 |
| Construction | 1 in 3,000 |
| 20 mSv radiation per year | 1 in 1,200 |
| Mining | 1 in 1,100 |
| Forestry | 1 in 900 |
| Fishing and Hunting | 1 in 500 |

**Note:** Includes deaths arising out of occupational illnesses, but does not include deaths among the 20% of all workers who were not covered by workers compensation. Data based on compilations by the Occupational Safety and Health Branch of Labour Canada.

about 34 years while the average loss due to a radiation induced cancer is about 13 years. Occupational hazards from radiation exposure at work will of course be added to the hazards from conventional accidents at work. This is a serious concern in uranium mines, where the rate of accidents is high, as it is in all other mining activities. On the other hand there have not been any fatal accidents during the operation of nuclear generating stations in Canada. Working in these nuclear stations, including the risk from radiation dose, could be considered a relatively safe occupation. If mining of fuels is excluded, the major occupational risk in all phases of the production and distribution of electricity is in the transmission and distribution of electricity. Electrical line workers may fall from poles or towers or be electrocuted, but there are no limits prescribed for this occupational risk. Continuing efforts are being made in our society to reduce all occupational hazards.

Acceptability of involuntary risks by members of the public is less clear and is a topic of continuing discussion. The ICRP has recommended a public dose limit of 1 mSv per year. The regulatory agency in Canada, the Atomic Energy Control Board (AECB), with the support of the ACRP, has indicated its intention to adopt this limit. However actual radiation doses received continue to be more

| AVERAGE ANNUAL RISK OF DEATH IN CANADA FROM FATAL ACCIDENTS OR FROM RADIATION EXPOSURE | |
|---|---|
| **Hazard** | **Risk of Death Per Year** |
| Accidents on the road | 1 in 5,000 |
| Accidents at home | 1 in 11,000 |
| Accidents at work | 1 in 24,000 |
| 1 mSv per year legal limit | 1 in 20,000 |
| 0.05 mSv per year maximum from nuclear facilities | 1 in 400,000 |
| 0.001 mSv per year average from nuclear facilities | 1 in 20,000,000 |

important than the legal limit. Utilities in Canada have set design and operating targets for the maximum radiation dose to members of the public from emissions during nuclear power station operation. The intent is to ensure that the annual dose to a member of the public is less than 0.05 mSv per year. The doses being achieved are below this value and are so low that the potential risks are well within acceptable standards for members of the public.

The public may also be exposed to radiation from waste materials resulting from the nuclear fuel cycle. The regulatory approach being taken by the AECB to disposal of radioactive waste in Canada is that the maximum radiation dose to any member of the public must be less than 0.05 mSv per year. As noted in the above table, potential health hazards at this dose level are very low.

There are important exceptions in applying dose limits. The limits do not apply to radiation exposures received:

- by patients in the course of medical diagnosis or treatment,

- by persons carrying out lifesaving procedures in an emergency, or

- by the public from natural sources.

For most medical diagnoses the potential personal benefits far outweigh the risk associated with the exposure. In some instances, for example in breast cancer detection using x-rays, an assessment has been carried out by the medical profession to show that the practice is justified for women more than 50 years of age. In addition, the medical profession has achieved considerable success in dose reduction in medical diagnosis and now considers this reduction a normal good practice.

All Canadians are exposed to natural sources of radiation. These background radiation levels are so low that any risk reduction achievable would be minor. Prescribing limits could be restrictive on personal freedom and enormously wasteful since time-consuming and expensive dose measurements would be required to show conformance to any limits established.

## RADIATION PROTECTION OF OTHER LIVING ORGANISMS

The ICRP has suggested that if individual humans are adequately protected against radiation exposure then other living species are also likely to be sufficiently protected. Extensive studies have been carried out on the effects of acute exposure of a wide variety of living organisms to high doses of radiation at high dose rates. These studies have shown that mammals, including humans, are generally the most sensitive to radiation. The range of lethal doses for different living organisms extends up to about 3,000 times that for humans. This applies to certain bacteria and primitive plants. Extensive field studies have also been carried out in Canada and the U.S.A. on the effects of chronic exposure of plants in their natural environment to gamma radiation at different dose rates.

These studies have confirmed that gamma rays at low dose rates are less damaging than at high dose rates. Even the most sensitive plants in the natural environment do not suffer any detectable harm with dose rates up to 1000 times higher than those which they normally receive from natural sources. There is no doubt that small increases in their normal exposure to radiation will not threaten the survival of these species in any way.

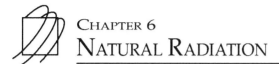

# CHAPTER 6
# NATURAL RADIATION

Radiation and radioactivity have been part of the earth's environment through all geological time. Ionizing radiation comes from the earth itself and sources beyond the earth. The latter comes from the sun and from outer space, and is called cosmic radiation. The cosmic radiation from outer space does not change much with time, but that from the sun changes intensity with the occurrence of solar flares. Cosmic radiation interacts with elements in the atmosphere to produce radionuclides such as tritium and carbon-14. These are called cosmogenic radionuclides because of their origin. Radiation from the earth itself comes from naturally occurring radionuclides in the rocks of the earth's surface. These are called primordial radionuclides since they were present when the earth was first formed. They include uranium, thorium and potassium. The radiation from them is primordial radiation (Figure 6.1).

## COSMIC RADIATION

Cosmic rays bend in the earth's magnetic field, so more enter near the poles than near the equator. They are also absorbed by the atmosphere so the intensity increases with height above sea level, roughly doubling for each increase in height of 1,800 metres. Buildings also absorb cosmic radiation so its intensity is lower indoors than outdoors. At sea level in the middle latitudes, the annual dose from cosmic radiation is about 0.3 mSv.

## COSMOGENIC RADIONUCLIDES

Many nuclides are produced by cosmic rays but only four, carbon-14, beryllium-7, sodium-22 and tritium (hydrogen-3) are important contributors to the radiation dose people receive. Together they contribute, by ingestion and subsequent internal irradiation of body organs and tissues, an annual dose of about 0.015 mSv. Carbon-14 contributes 80% of this total.

## PRIMORDIAL RADIONUCLIDES

Rocks, soils and all materials which contact them such as vegetables and water, contain potassium-40, uranium and thorium. All are radioactive. Uranium and thorium each have many decay products that are also radioactive. Potassium-40 occurs mixed with stable, non-radioactive potassium at a concentration of about 120 parts per million (ppm), i.e. in every million atoms of natural potassium there are 120 radioactive potassium-40 atoms. The rest are stable.

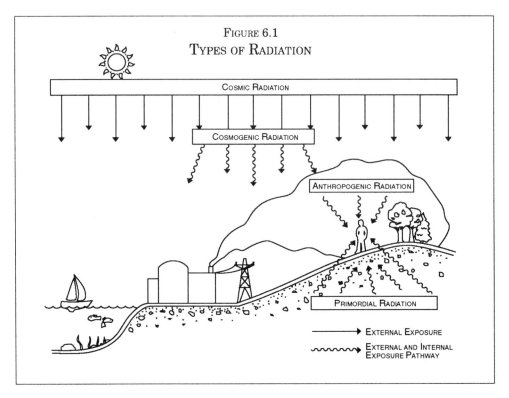

FIGURE 6.1
TYPES OF RADIATION

COSMIC RADIATION

COSMOGENIC RADIATION

ANTHROPOGENIC RADIATION

PRIMORDIAL RADIATION

→ EXTERNAL EXPOSURE

⟿ EXTERNAL AND INTERNAL EXPOSURE PATHWAY

The average concentration of uranium in rocks and soils is a few ppm, but much higher concentrations can occur in certain locations. When the concentration in ore exceeds a thousand ppm it may be economical to mine. Concentrations tend to be higher in igneous than in sedimentary rocks, and higher concentrations occur along the southern edge of the Canadian shield. Thorium is also widely though unevenly distributed. Both uranium and thorium are at the start of long chains of radioactive isotopes that end with stable, non-radioactive isotopes of lead. Of special importance among the two sets of decay products are the gases radon and thoron, of which more will be said later.

Primordial radionuclides are the source of external and internal exposure when they are ingested or inhaled and subsequently deposited in the body. Exposure to external radiation occurs not only outdoors but also indoors. This is because building materials contain primordial radionuclides. The doses to which people are exposed vary from place to place according to concentrations in soils and rocks and the building materials used in the construction of their homes. The average annual local dose is about 0.12 mSv from potassium-40, and 0.23 mSv from uranium and thorium and their decay products.

External radiation from primordial radionuclides adds to that from cosmic rays and the two are usually measured together. Measurements by Health Canada show that the average annual external dose in areas of 'normal' background in Canada is 0.65 mSv, about the same as the average for the rest of the world. It is more or less the same in all the larger centres of population across Canada. In the north-west around Whitehorse and Yellowknife it is slightly higher than average, and in the north-central part of the country around Moosonee and Churchill it is slightly lower. During the three or four months of winter, shielding provided by snow cover reduces the external dose rate outdoors from ground sources by nearly half. Similarly, snow cover reduces radon seepage from the soil.

Primordial radionuclides enter the body by several routes. Dusts containing these radionuclides may be blown into the air and inhaled; water which has drained through soils and rocks and dissolved these radionuclides may be a source of drinking water. Vegetables and animals which have absorbed these radionuclides are used as food.

How potassium-40 enters a person's body, or where the person lives, does not affect the dose received from this radionuclide. This is because the potassium-40 activity per unit weight of natural potassium is fixed and the amount of natural potassium in the body is constant; therefore the internal dose received is constant. For example, an average adult male has about 2 g of potassium for each kilogram of body weight and therefore about 60 Bq of potassium-40. From this he receives an annual dose of about 0.19 mSv.

In most places uranium and thorium enter the body by ingestion rather than by inhalation. Radioactivity and radiation levels are measured across the country by Health Canada routinely, and in periodic special surveys. The Canadian data quoted in this and later chapters come from reports published by this federal department. The amounts of uranium and thorium entering the body depend on where a person lives and obtains food and water. The concentration of uranium in surface drinking water in most areas is less than 1 mBq per litre, but in some areas much higher concentrations can be found, particularly when drinking water is obtained from wells. According to figures quoted in an UNSCEAR report of 1982, a concentration of 200 Bq per litre has been measured in drinking water from a well in Helsinki, Finland. In Regina, where some water is obtained from wells, the average concentration is about 150 mBq per litre.

Although both thorium and uranium have approximately the same concentration in soil, thorium is poorly absorbed by the digestive tract so that it is a less important contributor to human exposure than uranium. Radium-226, one of the decay products of uranium-238, can be an important contributor to internal dose. Food is normally more important as a source of radium-226 entering the body than inhalation, or drinking surface water. Well waters, however, may contain high concentrations of radium-226. In some parts of the world concentrations greater than 100 mBq of radium-226 per litre of well water have been found.

Levels as high as this have not been found in any drinking water in Canada. The highest occur at Elliot Lake and these are less than 20 mBq per litre. Measurements have been made of the radium-226 in drinking water in Ottawa, Port Hope and Regina. The concentration is less than 5 mBq per litre. At this level the average annual dose due to internal exposure from uranium and thorium and their decay products is about 0.04 mSv in Canada.

## RADON DECAY PRODUCTS

Radium decays to the radioactive gases radon and thoron which are much more mobile than uranium and thorium and their solid decay products like radium. Radon and thoron seep from the ground into the atmosphere where they are soon blown away by the wind. The resulting exposures are comparatively small. But the gases may also seep into houses, mostly through basement floors and walls. If building materials contain uranium or thorium then radon and thoron may also enter houses from this source. When these gases decay they form solid radioactive products which become attached to dust particles and may enter the body by inhalation and so expose the lungs. Inside buildings, they cannot be carried away by the wind so their concentrations and those of their decay products rise.

Concerns about radon and thoron have increased since improved building standards have been developed to conserve energy. As ventilation rates of homes have decreased, concentrations of radon and thoron decay products in homes have increased. In some locations in Canada, soil containing high concentrations of radium has been used to backfill excavations around basement walls. This has resulted in high concentrations of radon in the basements of these houses.

The radon level in buildings depends on how much radium is in the well water and in the rocks and soil around the building, on the type of material used for construction and on the building ventilation rate. More than 13,000 houses in 19 Canadian cities have been checked for concentrations of radon decay products. The average concentration of radon decay products was 17 $Bq/m^3$ which is estimated to give an effective dose of 1 mSv per year. However, the measurements were made in summer when houses are usually ventilated better than in winter, so it is likely the actual doses are higher. Large differences were found across the country but the differences within cities were usually larger.

Several places were also surveyed because they were suspected of having higher concentrations. In March Township near Ottawa, for example, concentrations in 343 houses were measured because uranium deposits found nearby had concentrations of 5 ppm uranium. More than half the houses had concentrations of radon decay products less than 19 $Bq/m^3$. The average was 50 $Bq/m^3$ and the highest was 700 $Bq/m^3$. An area in British Columbia was surveyed because high radon concentrations were found in water in the area. Nearly half the houses surveyed had concentrations of radon decay products less than 19 Bq/m$^3$. The average was 74 Bq/m$^3$ and the highest 2900 Bq/m$^3$.

There is no direct evidence that exposure to the levels of radon decay products found in homes has any harmful effects. However, Health Canada has established a guideline of 800 Bq/m$^3$ for the maximum level of radon in homes. Corrective action is recommended to reduce the radon level if this value is exceeded.

Concentrations of radon and its decay products may be reduced in a home by one or more methods. If the high concentrations have arisen because high radium-content material, from mines or tailings, has been used to backfill around basements, the material can be removed. Radon can also be prevented from entering homes by placing a barrier between the source and the interior of the home. Installation of underflow ventilation, for example weeping tiles below a basement floor exhausting to a duct or chimney, will divert radon and reduce the amount entering a home. The radon levels in a home can also be reduced by filtration of the air or the use of other air cleaning devices, or simply by increasing the number of ventilation air changes per hour. For this latter method some form of air-to-air heat exchanger must be installed to reduce heat loss from the home.

There is insufficient information to give a precise value for the average dose a person receives from radon daughter products in Canada. The dose rate from this source is subject to large variations across the country and even within cities. The value of 1 mSv per person per year has been adopted for the average effective dose from this source for this booklet, but there is considerable uncertainty in this value.

## TOTAL DOSES

The worldwide average total dose from radiation of natural origin is about 2 mSv per year. This value may be used for Canada but there will be parts of the country where the average dose will be higher, perhaps as high as 3 mSv per year.

| AVERAGE ANNUAL EFFECTIVE DOSE FROM RADIATION OF NATURAL ORIGIN ||
|---|---|
| **Sources** | **mSv** |
| External radiation | |
| Cosmic | 0.30 |
| Primordial | 0.35 |
| Total External | 0.65 |
| Internal Radiation | |
| Primordial | 0.35 |
| Cosmogenic | 0.01 |
| Radon | 1.0 |
| Thoron | 0.1 |
| Total Internal (rounded) | 1.5 |
| Total (rounded) | 2 |

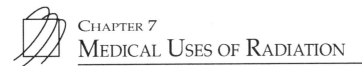

CHAPTER 7

# MEDICAL USES OF RADIATION

The largest source of exposure of Canadians to ionizing radiation after natural sources is the medical and dental use of x-rays and the medical use of radioactive materials. Radiation is used in medical practice in two ways, either to help diagnose illness or to kill cancerous cells (radiotherapy). In major industrialized countries, the average dose from medical uses of radiation is almost 1 mSv per year. This is equal to one half to one third of the average radiation dose from natural sources in most areas.

Diagnostic examination using x-rays contributes about 90% of the radiation dose the population receives from medical sources. In industrialized countries, the annual number of these examinations, including dental, ranges from 300 to nearly 2,000 per thousand inhabitants. The fraction of the total that is contributed by dental examination varies from 1% to 30%. In Canada, the number of diagnostic x-rays carried out annually is about 1,200 per thousand of the population, 14% of which come from dental x-rays.

A diagnostic procedure which is much less frequently used than x-rays is one in which a gamma emitting radionuclide is given internally to a patient so that the

| Examination | Percentage | |
| --- | --- | --- |
| | Of All Exams | Collective* Dose |
| Limbs | 22 | 0.9 |
| Chest | 25 | 1.7 |
| Dental | 13 | 0.4 |
| Spine | 9 | 14 |
| Head | 5 | 1 |
| Digestive tract | 9 | 43 |
| Abdomen | 2 | 4 |
| Urinary system | 2 | 12 |
| Others | 13 | 23 |

**X-RAY EXAMINATION IN CANADA PERCENTAGE BY TYPE AND CONTRIBUTION TO COLLECTIVE DOSE**

\* Estimate based on U.K. data for dose per type of examination

behaviour of the radionuclide in the patient can be followed and the functioning of an organ or flow of blood studied.

In most diagnostic procedures the doses are small. By contrast, in radiotherapy for the treatment of cancers the doses administered are large. Comparatively few patients receive this treatment; the patients are already in a life threatening situation and the radiation doses are intended to kill cancer cells. Doses to normal tissues are minimized.

## Diagnostic X-Rays

All materials absorb x-rays to varying degrees depending on their density and elemental composition. When they pass through the body, differences in the density and composition of the tissues they go through result in varying degrees of darkening of an x-ray film placed behind the patient. Bone is particularly dense and shows up distinctly so that cracks and breaks can be easily spotted. When interpreted by a specialist, more subtle changes in other tissues can give clues to the presence of disease.

Nearly 31 million radiological examinations are carried out yearly in Canada, almost one a year per person. Chest radiographs account for about 26% of the total, followed by x-rays of the shoulder, pelvis and limbs, which account for another 22%. These along with dental x-ray examinations are estimated to make up about 60% of the total. These examinations involve relatively low doses, typically about 0.02 mSv for a dental examination; recent measurements suggest that the average dose from a diagnostic chest x-ray in Canada is about 0.07 mSv.

Much larger doses are associated with examinations of the digestive and urinary tracts, both of which involve multiple exposures and the administration of contrast agents to outline the soft tissues. Doses received by patients in these examinations may be as much as 1 mSv.

X-ray examinations of the spine account for about nine percent of all diagnostic examinations in Canada. Doses are lower than for digestive tract procedures but higher than for chest x-rays.

| APPROXIMATE ANNUAL NUMBER OF DIAGNOSTIC X-RAYS IN CANADA |
| --- |
| 31 Million |

Although the number of x-ray examinations carried out has increased significantly in recent years, the doses integrated over the population have tended to decrease because of improvements to x-ray machines and improved procedures.

Nevertheless, measurements made in Britain in 1983/84 show large differences, up to a factor of 100 between the highest and lowest doses for the same examination depending on where it is carried out. Similar large differences probably exist elsewhere, including Canada. Even at the same medical facility the dose associated with a given examination can differ from patient to patient because of their individual needs. Average doses per person from diagnostic x-ray examinations also differ from one country to another, as may be seen from the table on the next page.

These measurements are difficult and expensive to carry out. Methods used differ from one study to another even in the same country, and may produce different

| AVERAGE ANNUAL DOSE FROM X-RAYS IN VARIOUS COUNTRIES | | | |
|---|---|---|---|
| Country | Dose (mSv) | Country | Dose (mSv) |
| Poland | 1.7 | Italy | 0.8 |
| France | 1.6 | Spain | 0.8 |
| USSR | 1.4 | Finland | 0.7 |
| Japan | 1.3 | Sweden | 0.6 |
| USA | 1.3 | United Kingdom | 0.2 |

results. The estimated average dose from diagnostic x-rays per person in Canada is about 0.6 mSv, and this is low among the estimates from countries having similar levels of medical attention, i.e. less than 1,000 patients per physician. The figure for Canada may well be higher, perhaps close to the value given in the table for the U.S.A. The important point is that, even for the United Kingdom, the dose from medical diagnostic x-ray examinations is much larger than the dose from any other man-made radiation source. It is therefore important that exposures from this source be kept as low as practicable, consistent with obtaining acceptable image quality. Much has been done and continues to be done to lower doses per examination by improving techniques and equipment.

| ANNUAL DOSE FROM DIAGNOSTIC X-RAY EXAMINATIONS IN CANADA | |
|---|---|
| Collective Dose | 16,200 person·Sv |
| Average Individual Dose | 0.6 mSv |

## COMPUTED TOMOGRAPHY

A technique involving body scanners and computed tomography (CT) was introduced in the 1970s and its use has steadily increased since. In this, an x-ray source rotates around the patient and is measured by a row of detectors after it has passed through the patient's body. Many measurements are made and the results fed to a computer which reconstructs an image of a cross-section of the patient. Unlike conventional x-ray examinations which sum all the effects of differentially absorbing tissues along the beam path, CT builds up a picture of those effects separately in a thin cross-section of the body.

Within ten years of its introduction, over 2,000 scanners were in use in the U.S.A. alone and the number was increasing at the rate of about 200 units per year. In Manitoba, the number of scans carried out in 1977 was 0.85 per 1,000 of population. By 1980 this had reached 4.6 scans per 1,000 of population and by 1987, 18.2. The trend was the same in Quebec, where the number of scans rose from 1.4 per 1,000 population in 1977 to nearly 10 per 1,000 population in 1988.

In Manitoba, the average dose per year per person rose from 0.0007 mSv in 1977 to 0.081 mSv in 1987. The increase was due to the nearly five-fold increase in the numbers of people scanned, and a similar increase in the dose per scan. The dose per scan in Manitoba increased from a little less than 1 mSv to about 45 mSv in the period form 1977 to 1987. It has been projected that the number of examinations will eventually reach 28 per thousand, and the average dose per person at that time will be 0.12 mSv per year. Computed tomography will join diagnostic procedures such as barium enemas which now contribute significantly to the population dose from diagnostic x-ray examination.

Applications of physical devices and techniques to medical diagnostic procedures is rapidly changing as new technologies are introduced and older ones find wider applications. Not all these new technologies involve radiation and some of these are already replacing radiological techniques. For example, the use of ultrasound as a diagnostic tool has increased sharply and has begun to replace conventional x-ray procedures in urinary tract and other examinations. The distribution and size of medical exposure is expected to change significantly in the next few decades.

## NUCLEAR MEDICINE

In nuclear medicine, the patient receives, either by intravenous injection or by mouth, a drug into which a gamma-ray-emitting radionuclide has been incorporated. The drug is one chosen to be taken up preferentially by a particular organ or tissue whose functioning is to be assessed. The distribution of the drug is then followed by scanning the patient with a gamma camera. Sometimes the radioactive drug can be used in treatment, e.g. thyroid disease.

Applications of nuclear medicine have been increasing rapidly over the last 20 years, though in terms of number of examinations these still lag far behind diagnostic x-rays. Many hundreds of diagnostic x-rays are taken per 1,000 of the population but examinations by nuclear medicine procedures are in the tens per 1,000 of population.

The radionuclide technetium-99m is the one most frequently used in diagnostic radionuclide procedures. Bound to a suitable compound, it is used to diagnose illnesses and malfunctions of the brain, bone, liver and kidney, and for assessing blood flow. Technetium-99m results from the beta decay of molybdenum-99, the world supply of which is largely produced in a Canadian reactor at Chalk River.

## RADIOTHERAPY

Radiotherapy is the treatment of cancer by killing tumour cells using beams of high energy gamma-rays from the radionuclide cobalt-60 or from accelerators. Some tumours may also be treated by inserting radioactive sources into the body beside the tumour, using specially shaped applicators.

Canada is a major supplier of cobalt-60, cobalt-60 therapy units and accelerators. The aim of the treatment is to deliver a high dose to the tumour but as little dose as possible to the surrounding healthy tissue. Consequently a large source, providing a narrow beam of high energy radiation, is rotated around the patient. The pattern and properties of the beam are carefully worked out by the hospital physicist on a case by case basis to maximize the destruction of the tumour and avoid complications from irradiation of healthy tissue. Nonetheless, the treatment is drastic and accompanied by unpleasant side-effects.

Radioactive sources emitting beta radiation are useful for treating shallow tumours, such as skin tumours. The advantage is that very little of the deep tissue underlying the tumour is irradiated.

## CONTROLLING DIAGNOSTIC MEDICAL EXPOSURES

Medical exposures differ from other man-made sources of radiation exposure in that they are to some extent controlled personally by the patient acting on information about the risks and expected benefits supplied by a medical advisor from his or her knowledge of the patient's physical and mental condition. Outside intervention by legislating generalized

dose limits is therefore not appropriate. Nevertheless, the other principles of radiation protection apply. The radiation dose that will be received and its attendant risks must be justified by the expected benefits; other, safer procedures of at least equal merit must not be available; and the dose must be as low as is reasonably achievable, consistent with obtaining the desired medical result. Application of these principles is obviously important to the patient, and because of the relatively large population doses, to society. Using data from the United Kingdom for the dose per examination by type, and the number of examinations of each type performed in Canada, an estimate may be made of the average dose per person in Canada. This is about 0.6 mSv per year, compared to 0.28 mSv in the United Kingdom and about 0.6 mSv in the U.S.A. Nearly three quarters of the Canadian total comes from diagnostic x-rays of the digestive tract and gall bladder.

Since diagnostic x-rays are responsible for most of the collective dose, it is important to continue efforts to reduce these. Keeping individual exposures low, without loss of beneficial diagnostic accuracy and results, requires constant attention from physicians and radiographers. Equipment must be properly adjusted and maintained and efforts to keep the beam within the target area must be pursued to the highest standards. No more patient exposures should be carried out than are absolutely necessary. The patient has a right to question duplication of x-ray examinations.

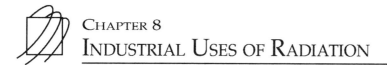

# Chapter 8

# Industrial Uses of Radiation

Medical uses of radiation provide important human benefits but there are also important and beneficial industrial uses. In Canada there are about 3,000 radioisotope licences for industrial and scientific uses of radioactive materials. The uses depend upon the unique characteristics of ionizing radiation. For the most part, these can be classified into three main groupings: uses which depend upon the penetrating ability of radiation; uses which involve neutron sources and the ability of neutrons to make materials radioactive; and uses which depend upon the ability of ionizing radiation to destroy or damage biological materials in some way.

In the first of these groups are industrial radiography, measurements using level gauges, and industrial thickness gauges. The second group includes well-logging, and methods for the detection and analysis of trace quantities of elements in biological and environmental materials. In the third and last group are techniques to sterilize medical equipment, preserve food and eradicate insect pests. There are some other uses such as in smoke detectors, static eliminators and emergency lighting which depend on other unique characteristics of radiation.

## Industrial Radiography

Industrial radiography is a process similar to the taking of medical x-rays, except that shadow films are taken of inanimate objects, instead of parts of the body. X-ray machines are sometimes used in fixed installations but more often gamma emitting sources are used in portable equipment.

A very simple device is shown in Figures 8.1A and 8.1B. In this device a source within the shielded container can be rotated from a shielded position (Figure 8.1A) to a position where it emits a beam of gamma rays. The image produced on a film placed behind an object in the beam is dependent on the thickness and density of the object (Figure 8.1B). Defects in the object such as voids or cracks may be seen on the film. Radiography cameras of this design are not licensed in Canada although they are used in other countries. It has been described because it provides a simple illustration of the principle of industrial gamma radiography.

The type and strength of the gamma source used depends on the mass of the object and the material of which it is composed. Sources which emit high energy gamma radiation are used for massive, dense objects, and sources which emit low energy gamma rays are used for light, thin objects.

INDUSTRIAL GAMMA-RAY SOURCES AND THEIR APPLICATIONS

| Source | Application & Thickness Limits |
|--------|-------------------------------|
| Thulium-170 | 0.25 cm to 1.5 cm plastics, wood, light alloys, steel or equivalent. |
| Iridium-192 | 1 cm to 6 cm steel or equivalent. |
| Cesium-137 | 2.5 cm to 8 cm steel or equivalent. |
| Cobalt-60 | 6 cm to 22 cm steel or equivalent. |

Iridium-192 is commonly used, as it is suitable for taking films of the welds and valves in industrial piping in refineries, gas and water utilities, power stations, heating plants, etc. For this application, equipment known as a 'crank-out camera' is in wide use. This consists of a shielded container which houses a source that may be propelled along a guide tube using a crank and a long cable. When the crank is turned, the source is moved along the guide tube to a predetermined position, such as inside a pipe beside a weld. A strip of film placed around the weld will provide a radiograph of the weld and reveal any defects (Figure 8.2). The radiographer operating the equipment can stand well back from the source and so receives very little dose during the operations.

More than 140 companies are licensed to carry out radiography in Canada. Welds, joints, valves, etc., in industrial establishments are examined by this non-destructive process. This helps to produce high quality piping systems free of defects, and reduce the likelihood of failures with potentially serious consequences.

Throughout the world there have been some very bad accidents involving radiographic sources. The conditions and working environment of typical radiog-

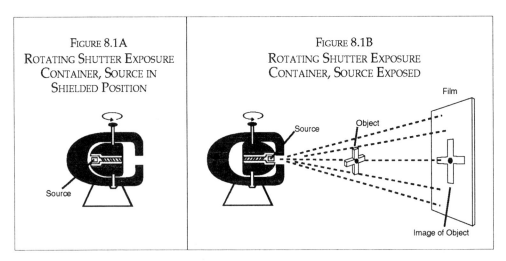

FIGURE 8.1A
ROTATING SHUTTER EXPOSURE CONTAINER, SOURCE IN SHIELDED POSITION

Source

FIGURE 8.1B
ROTATING SHUTTER EXPOSURE CONTAINER, SOURCE EXPOSED

Film

Source   Object

Image of Object

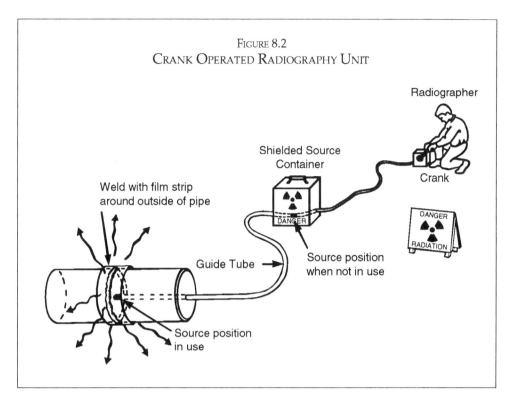

FIGURE 8.2
CRANK OPERATED RADIOGRAPHY UNIT

Radiographer

Shielded Source
Container

Crank

Weld with film strip
around outside of pipe

DANGER

DANGER
RADIATION

Guide Tube

Source position
when not in use

Source position
in use

raphy sites and projects appear to make accidents more probable than in others where radiation is used. A high level of regulatory attention is necessary to ensure satisfactory levels of safety in radiography work.

## NUCLEAR GAUGES

Modern production methods, especially automatic processes, require methods to monitor the quality of the products produced, or to control the process. Monitoring and control is often carried out by devices which use radioactive sources and the

unique ability of the radiation to penetrate materials. Figure 8.3 shows a gauge controlling the high and low levels of liquid in a tank.

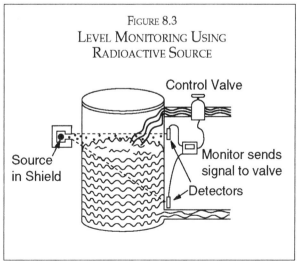

FIGURE 8.3
LEVEL MONITORING USING
RADIOACTIVE SOURCE

Control Valve

Source
in Shield

Monitor sends
signal to valve

Detectors

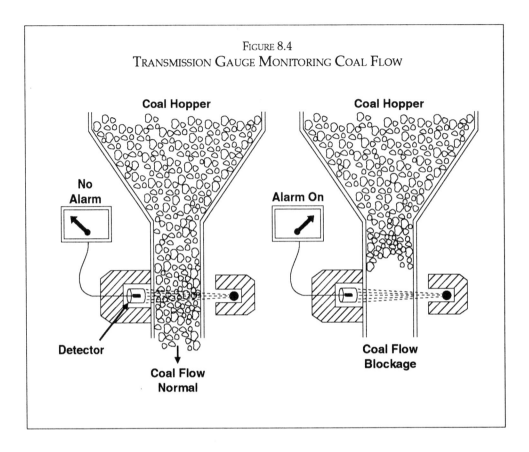

FIGURE 8.4
TRANSMISSION GAUGE MONITORING COAL FLOW

Coal Hopper

No Alarm

Detector

Coal Flow
Normal

Coal Hopper

Alarm On

Coal Flow
Blockage

Level gauges using radioactive sources have advantages over other types of gauges. They do not need to be in contact with the material being controlled or examined and so can be used on high speed processes, and on materials with extreme temperatures or harmful chemical properties.

Another useful application of this type of gauge is to monitor flow of material in a pipe or chute. In coal fired generating stations the flow of coal into the furnace is monitored in this way (Figure 8.4). If a blockage occurs, an alarm allows action to be taken to remove the blockage.

Portable versions of gauges using the principle of absorption of radiation are used to measure the density of soil. In its simplest form, a gamma ray source is placed in a hole in the ground. A detector, in another nearby hole, or at the surface, gives a reading which is dependent on the density of the soil (Figure 8.5).

Soil density may also be estimated by measuring the radiation which is reflected or 'backscattered' from the soil (Figure 8.6). High density materials backscatter more radiation than low density materials so the gauge can be calibrated to read soil density. Portable gauges of this type, using neutron emitting sources and neutron detectors, can be used to measure

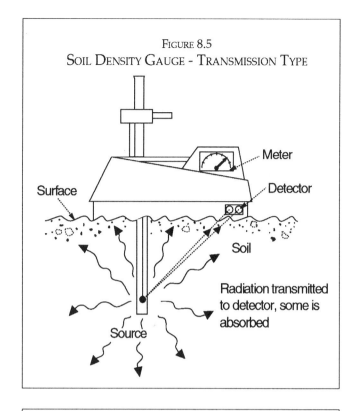

FIGURE 8.5
SOIL DENSITY GAUGE - TRANSMISSION TYPE

Meter

Surface

Detector

Soil

Radiation transmitted
to detector, some is
absorbed

Source

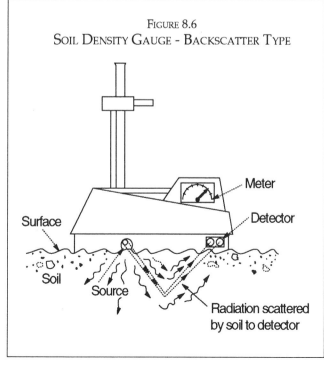

FIGURE 8.6
SOIL DENSITY GAUGE - BACKSCATTER TYPE

Meter

Surface

Detector

Soil

Source

Radiation scattered
by soil to detector

soil moisture content. Neutrons are very effectively backscattered by hydrogen atoms in water molecules.

Soil moisture and density gauges have been in use for over 40 years for measurements in civil engineering, agriculture and hydrology. For example, civil engineers will use these devices to establish how the soil will deform under loads or how much it has been compacted. In agriculture, estimates can be obtained of moisture content to predict crop yields; and in hydrology, the amount of water being consumed by plants and evaporation may be estimated. All these devices are constructed to strict standards which, along with the licensing requirements of the AECB, provide a high degree of assurance of safe operation. Measurements of the doses received by operators of these gauges show that these are less than 1 mSv per year.

Devices using beta sources are effective in

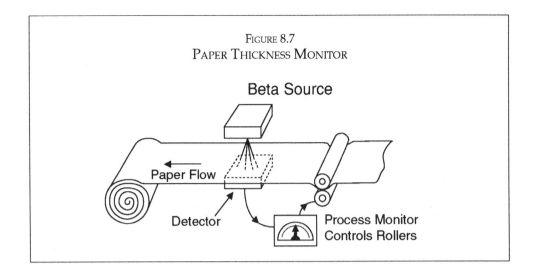

FIGURE 8.7
PAPER THICKNESS MONITOR

Beta Source

Paper Flow

Detector

Process Monitor
Controls Rollers

controlling the thickness of plastic or paper during production. Low energy beta radiation is absorbed readily by thin films of such materials. A detector and low energy beta source are placed on opposite sides of paper sheet emerging from the production machines. If the paper thickness begins to decrease from the desired value, the signal from the detector increases, and the process monitor moves the rollers apart. The opposite effect occurs if the paper thickness increases, (Figure 8.7).

## NEUTRON ACTIVATION ANALYSIS

Neutron activation analysis is a powerful process for determining the constituent elements in materials. Neutrons may interact with the atoms of elements in a variety of ways. One of these is known as a neutron-gamma reaction. This is usually written $(n,\gamma)$ reaction. Typically what occurs in an $(n,\gamma)$ reaction is shown in Figure 8.8.

A neutron from a source of some kind hits a target nucleus and forms a compound nucleus which promptly emits a gamma ray, known as a *prompt gamma ray*. Atoms which remain after the emission of the prompt gamma rays are still unstable, i.e. radioactive, and they usually undergo radioactive decay with the emission of a beta ray and a gamma ray. The neutron activation analysis method relies on the measurement of the energy of either the prompt gamma ray or the radioactive decay gamma ray. The energy of these gamma rays is characteristic of the target nucleus, which can therefore be uniquely identified. The method using prompt gamma rays can be used for on-line or continuous measurement. The method using the radioactive decay nucleus is generally used in a batch or single sample process. For some elements, very small amounts may be measured by this technique.

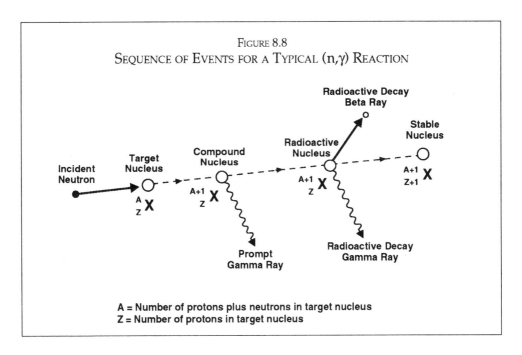

FIGURE 8.8
SEQUENCE OF EVENTS FOR A TYPICAL $(n,\gamma)$ REACTION

A = Number of protons plus neutrons in target nucleus
Z = Number of protons in target nucleus

The accompanying table gives detection limits using batch analysis that can readily be achieved for some elements. These levels can be measured simultaneously, in a one gram sample, without chemical treatment of the sample. Much lower levels may be detected if chemical analysis is used and the sample size and neutron flux are increased. For example, levels of copper as low as 0.1 billionth of a gram ($10^{-13}$ g) per gram of sample may be measured.

### TYPICAL DETECTION LIMITS IN 1 g SAMPLE OF ROCK USING NEUTRON ACTIVATION ANALYSIS

| Element | Detection Limit ($\mu$g) |
|---------|--------------------------|
| Cobalt | 0.1 |
| Chromium | 0.5 |
| Arsenic | 1 |
| Gold | 2 |
| Zinc | 10 |
| Nickel | 50 |

Neutron activation analysis is used in archaeology, environmental science, geology, medicine, forensic science and industry generally. In environmental science, trace contaminants such as copper can be measured in animals, birds, fish, food, ground water, rain, and plants to very low levels. Even for lead, it is possible to measure ten millionths of a gram in a sample. Besides being very sensitive, neutron activation analysis has the advantage that as many as 30 elements may be measured simultaneously in a very small sample without destroying the sample.

In on-line analysis the energies of the prompt gamma rays emitted when a substance is bombarded by neutrons are measured, (see Figure 8.8). The energies of the gamma rays emitted are characteristic of the target atom. This enables the target atom to be identified and the quantity present to be estimated.

A typical use is to measure the concentration of elements in ores, coal, cement or raw glass mixtures. A small sample stream is taken from the main conveyor stream. This sample stream is exposed to a beam of neutrons from a neutron source and the elements in the ore or coal are identified by the prompt gamma rays emitted. A schematic of a typical coal analyzer is shown in Figure 8.9.

The process can be used for monitoring coal quality, blending or sorting of the coal.

Another application of neutron-activation is in well-logging, particularly of oil wells. Companies drilling wells for oil or water need information on the strata of rocks through which they are drilling, and the oil and water content of the strata.

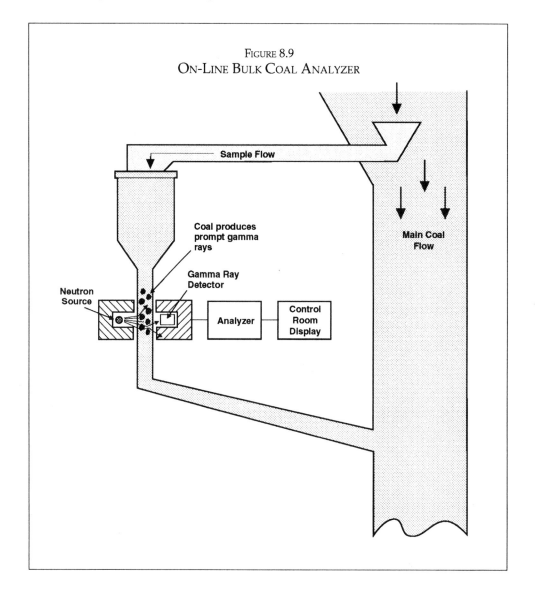

FIGURE 8.9
ON-LINE BULK COAL ANALYZER

Well-logging using gamma and neutron sources provides the information needed. A probe containing a neutron source and a gamma ray detector is passed down the borehole. Measurement of prompt gamma radiation, characteristic of the materials encountered, identifies the elements in the rock the detector is passing through. Well-logging also uses the back-scattering of radiation described previously for portable gauges. Gamma radiation sources used in this way provide information on the rock type. If a neutron detector is added to the probe, then when used with a neutron emitting source, information can be obtained on the oil or water content of the rock. The arrangement of detector and source is shown in Figure 8.10.

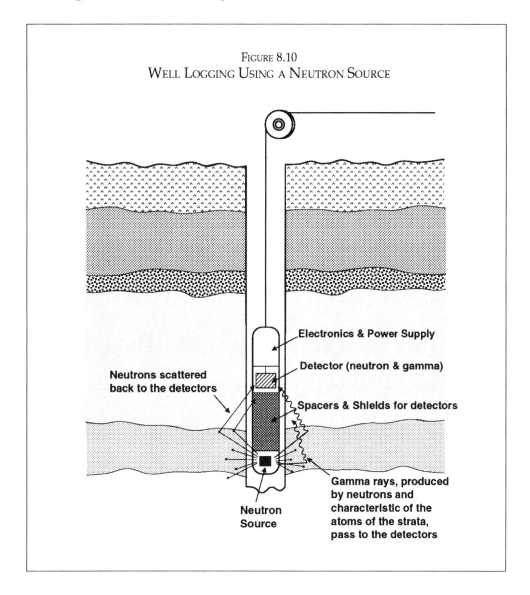

FIGURE 8.10
WELL LOGGING USING A NEUTRON SOURCE

Electronics & Power Supply

Detector (neutron & gamma)

Neutrons scattered
back to the detectors

Spacers & Shields for detectors

Gamma rays, produced
by neutrons and
characteristic of the
atoms of the strata,
pass to the detectors

Neutron
Source

As the source and detector descends the well, information is recorded at the well-head. The information is correlated with the depth of the hole. This enables the oil company engineers or hydrologists boring the hole to make estimates of oil or water content, and therefore the potential resources of these liquids.

## STERILIZATION OF MEDICAL PRODUCTS

The critical need for sterilization of medical instruments and products has been understood for over 100 years. The work of Lord Joseph Lister highlighted this and resulted in a reduced incidence of postoperative infections. With the acceptance of the germ theory of disease, various methods of sterilization evolved, such as use of chemicals, steam sterilization, and dry heat.

Sterilization using ionizing radiation was first introduced commercially in Scotland in 1957. This technique has several advantages over some of the traditional older techniques. For example, prolonged exposure to high temperatures may destroy or damage some plastics. Steam exposure may dissolve some substances.

Sterilization by using ionizing radiation is simple in principle. The medical equipment or products are exposed to very high doses of gamma radiation, x-rays or high energy electrons. Gamma rays from cobalt-60 are now generally employed, and a dose of about 10 kGy delivered to the products will provide sterility safety equal to that of other methods. Because of the penetrating ability of gamma radiation, products such as hypodermic materials, fluid tubing and sutures may be prepacked in plastic or a metal-foil sealed container and subsequently sterilized. The process is particularly useful for absorbable sutures which are quite difficult to sterilize by other techniques.

## FOOD PRESERVATION BY IRRADIATION

Another rapidly growing technology, based on the ability of ionizing radiation in high doses to destroy living organisms, is food preservation. Food-transmitted infections are a source of serious health problems in nearly all parts of the world, especially third world countries. Even advanced countries suffer from such diseases, particularly those spread by food of animal origin carrying agents such as salmonella. The resultant costs to society are high.

Again the principle is simple and was first tested as early as 1916 in Sweden using x-rays. The food is irradiated to high doses between 5 and 10 kGy. This is sufficient to eliminate the contaminating agents. This technique of preservation and improving the safety of foodstuffs has advantages over other more conventional methods. At the dose levels used there is no induced toxicity or mutagenicity, the freshness and taste for most foods are not changed significantly, the food may be preserved after packaging, and the keeping quality is greatly improved. High doses of irradiation can affect the taste of some foods, so the dose must be carefully controlled for each specific food. A wide variety of foods have been processed in this way. Nordion International Inc. in Canada has been engaged in research in this area. It was shown at an early date that potatoes after irradiation would keep much better than untreated potatoes. Studies of this method of food preservation have shown significant reduction of infectious agents on many kinds of meat, fish, vegetables and fruits.

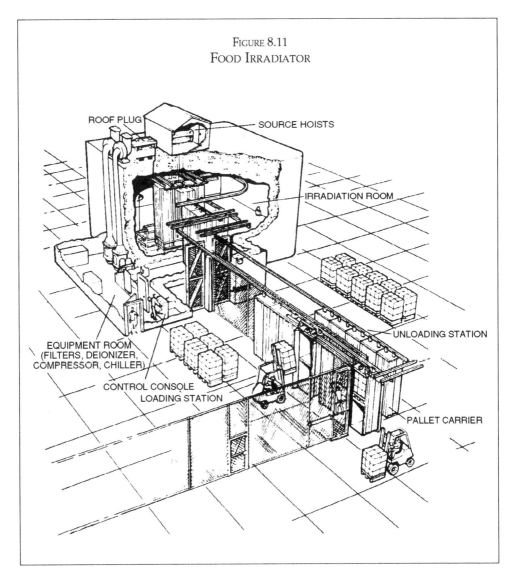

FIGURE 8.11
FOOD IRRADIATOR

A typical food irradiator includes a shielded source of radiation, an automated conveyor to move materials through the irradiation chamber, pre-treatment-rooms for chilling or freezing prior to irradiation, and packaging and storage rooms. An irradiator designed by Nordion International Inc. to irradiate pallets of food is shown in Figure 8.11.

There has been some public resistance to the use of radiation to preserve food. Several concerns have been expressed. One is that the food might itself be made radioactive. This does not happen if the gamma radiation used has an energy less than 10 Mev. Another concern is that the process might produce harmful toxins in the food. Compounds produced when ionizing radiation interacts with food molecules have not been found to impart toxic qualities to food. A number of agencies including the World Health Organization have fully endorsed food irradiation conducted under prescribed conditions.

Companies in the Netherlands, Norway, France, Belgium, Japan, South Africa and the U.S.A. are carrying out commercial preservation of food using radiation. Cobalt-60, provided mainly by Canada from Ontario Hydro nuclear power stations, is used in many irradiators throughout the world.

## CONTROL OF INSECT PESTS USING RADIATION STERILIZATION

The sterile insect technique has emerged in recent years as an important approach to biological control of insect pests. It was developed in the United States in the early 1950s and was first used successfully on the island of Curacao to eradicate the screwworm fly. This fly, which is about twice the size of a common housefly, attacks living animals, laying its eggs in open wounds such as scratches from barbed wire. When the eggs hatch into larvae these invade the wound and feed on the flesh of the animal. As the wound size increases, additional screwworm flies are attracted to it. Multiple infestations by the larvae of screwworms lead to sickness and frequently death of the animals. The screwworm fly was the cause of enormous losses to cattle farmers in the south of the United States and the sterile insect technique was developed to counteract this pest. The process is quite simple in principle. Large numbers of flies are raised in captivity and as pupae are exposed to about 100 Gy of gamma radiation. This does not prevent their development into active flies but does make them sexually sterile. When the flies hatch, they are released in large numbers (billions) in the infested areas. The sterile males swamp the natural males and compete to mate with natural females. The female flies mate only once and, if they have mated with a sterile male, lay eggs which do not hatch.

Success of this technique against an insect pest depends on two factors:

- the insect must be capable of being raised in large numbers in captivity

- females must mate only once

The screwworm meets these requirements.

The screwworm fly program has been remarkably successful and has resulted in the eradication of this pest in the United States and Northern Mexico. More recently, the technique was used to eradicate successfully an infestation of screwworm flies in Libya. The fly was apparently introduced by contaminated livestock and presented an enormous potential threat to African animals.

Unfortunately, the technique cannot be used against all insect pests because of the need to be able to raise the insects in captivity, and the requirement that the female only mate once. However it has been successful in eradicating the melon fly from the island of Rota and has been successful against the Mediterranean fruit fly in Costa Rica and Tunisia.

The sterile insect technique is being tested against other insects – the tsetse fly, cherry fruit fly, olive fly and onion fly. All these insect pests cause large commercial losses to farmers. Success against the tsetse fly would contribute greatly to improvements in the economies of many African countries. Pilot projects have been carried out successfully in Nigeria and Burkina Faso.

Canada, as a major supplier of cobalt-60 for irradiation facilities to sterilize these insects, is playing an important role in these projects.

## SMOKE DETECTORS

Canada ranks near the top of western countries in fire deaths per year (Figure 8.12), so that any device which contributes to a reduction in this risk is important in fire safety. The smoke detector is a modern device which is considered so effective in saving lives that some municipalities in Canada require that these be installed in all new homes.

One smoke detector type makes use of radioactive material and the properties of ionizing radiation. This detector, known as the Ionization Chamber Smoke Detector, is installed in many homes because it provides high reliability at low initial purchase and subsequent operating costs.

The operating principle of this type of detector depends on the ability of ionizing radiation to interact with atoms or molecules of a gas and detach electrons. If this is done in a confined space, such as between two metal plates, and a voltage is applied across the plates, (this is called an *ionization chamber*) the electrons will be collected at the positive plate as a tiny electric current (Figure 8.13).

FIGURE 8.12
FIRE DEATHS IN VARIOUS COUNTRIES

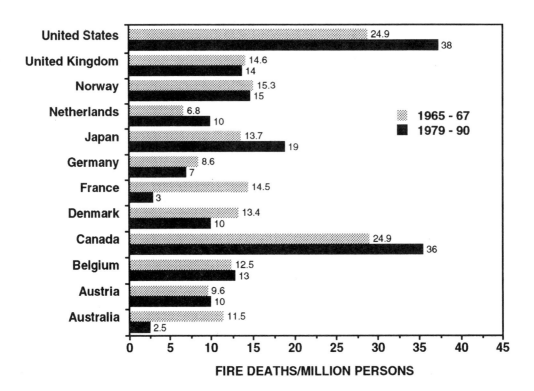

FIRE DEATHS/MILLION PERSONS

When the space between the plates is filled with a gas other than air, because of the difference in properties between this new gas and air, the electric current will be different – either smaller or larger. Smoke and other gases from fires will reduce the electric current substantially in a device like this. A typical ionization chamber smoke detector consists of two ionization chambers of equal volume sharing an alpha emitting radioactive source, Figure 8.14. One of the chambers contains clean air. The other has openings to allow room air to enter. Voltage is applied from batteries across the ionization chambers. When both chambers contain clean air, the current from the chambers is equal. When smoke and combustion gases enter the open chamber, the current from this chamber is reduced. A detector rapidly senses this difference in current from the two chambers, and triggers an audible alarm. It has been estimated that if early warning devices like this were installed in all homes then the number of deaths from fires could be reduced by 40 to 50%.

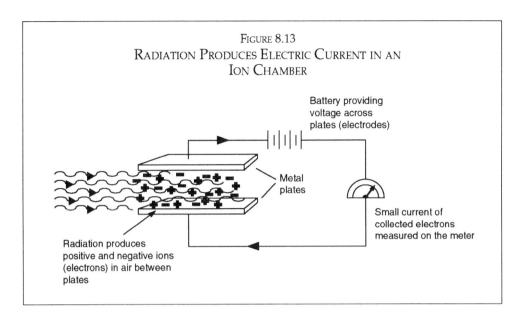

FIGURE 8.13
RADIATION PRODUCES ELECTRIC CURRENT IN AN
ION CHAMBER

Battery providing
voltage across
plates (electrodes)

Metal
plates

Small current of
collected electrons
measured on the meter

Radiation produces
positive and negative ions
(electrons) in air between
plates

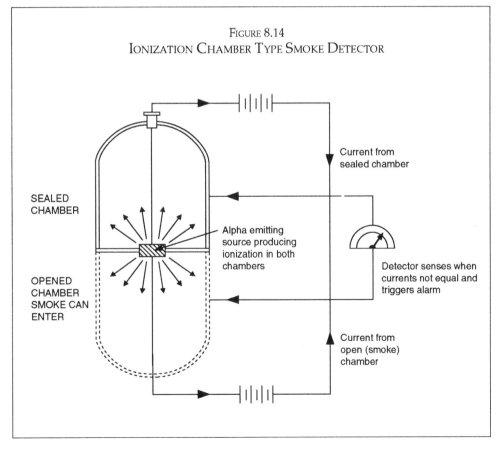

FIGURE 8.14
IONIZATION CHAMBER TYPE SMOKE DETECTOR

Current from
sealed chamber

SEALED
CHAMBER

Alpha emitting
source producing
ionization in both
chambers

Detector senses when
currents not equal and
triggers alarm

OPENED
CHAMBER
SMOKE CAN
ENTER

Current from
open (smoke)
chamber

## Radioactive Tracer Techniques

*Tracer technique* is the term applied to injecting a chemical into a process or an environmental system and following its flow or path through the system to understand what is happening to the chemical and to understand the system. Radioactive chemicals are particularly useful in this process because they can be readily detected and measured at very low levels.

The radioactive substance need not be man-made and many of the most useful studies, especially of environmental systems and of pollution, use naturally occurring radionuclides. Radioactive tracer techniques have been used to study ground water contamination, ocean circulation, sedimentation rates and the behaviour of the atmosphere.

## Miscellaneous Other Uses

There are many other uses of radionuclides including the provision of power for emergency light sources, some of which use tritium produced in CANDU reactors, and elimination of static electricity. Radioactive sources are also used in various ways in scientific instruments and dewpoint meters. There are also many specific applications in scientific research.

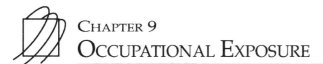

## CHAPTER 9
# OCCUPATIONAL EXPOSURE

There are many occupations in which exposure to ionizing radiation occurs. Approximately one in 100 Canadian workers is classified as a radiation worker. The obvious examples are those engaged in activities that produce or use radiation or radioactive material – industrial radiographers, nuclear station workers, and hospital employees who operate diagnostic x-ray machines and radiotherapy machines for cancer treatment.

In some occupations, exposure to natural sources of ionizing radiation occurs. Many miners are exposed as a result of the small quantities of uranium, thorium and potassium-40 present in various types of rock. The exposure is from two sources, gamma radiation and radon decay products. Gamma radiation is emitted by potassium-40 and the many radionuclides in the natural uranium and thorium decay chains. Radon decay products come primarily from radon-222 produced in the uranium-238 decay chain. This gas escapes into the mine from the walls and from crushed ores. Radon-222 itself is comparatively harmless but it decays very rapidly to alpha-particle-emitting radionuclides which attach themselves to dust particles in the mine atmosphere. When these are inhaled they irradiate the lungs.

Rather surprisingly in some occupations the doses received from natural sources are fairly high. Examples are workers producing potash-based fertilizer who are exposed to naturally occurring uranium, thorium and potassium-40 in the potash ores; and aircrew flying at high altitudes, around 10,000 metres, who are exposed to high levels of cosmic radiation.

## NATIONAL DOSE REGISTRY

Workers in Canada who are occupationally exposed to ionizing radiation from radioactive materials or x-rays, may be required to wear dose measuring devices (dosimeters), to measure the dose they receive at work, (Figure 9.1). The dosimeters are provided and measured by a certified dosimetry service.

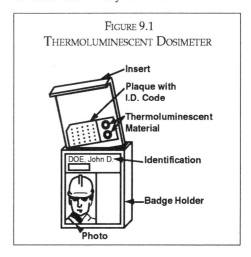

FIGURE 9.1
THERMOLUMINESCENT DOSIMETER

Insert
Plaque with I.D. Code
Thermoluminescent Material
DOE, John D. — Identification
Badge Holder
Photo

All occupational doses measured, regardless of who makes the measurement, are retained in the National Dose Registry managed by Health Canada. Occupational doses are measured and records retained for three main purposes:

- to demonstrate compliance with statutory dose limits and to assist in deciding whether doses are as low as reasonably achievable;
- to provide information for decisions on Workers' Compensation Board awards; and
- to provide a database which may be useful in refining estimates of the risk due to exposure to ionizing radiation.

It is a rare occurrence for radiation workers in Canada to exceed annual dose limits. There are about 110,000 workers whose radiation exposure is monitored regularly. Of this number less than one in 10,000 exceed the current annual dose limit of 50 mSv in the average year.

An annual report is prepared by Health Canada of the occupational doses received by job category.

In the 1970s the highest average annual doses were received by nuclear station workers but these are now much lower (Figure 9.2). This reduction has been achieved through improved designs and operating practices. Industrial radiographers now receive the highest average annual dose and have the highest incidence of workers exceeding occupational dose limits.

| AVERAGE* ANNUAL DOSES FOR VARIOUS OCCUPATIONS CANADA 1991 | |
|---|---|
| Occupation | Dose (mSv) |
| Dentist | 0.31 |
| Physician | 0.73 |
| Nurse | 0.40 |
| Veterinarian | 0.42 |
| Isotope Technician | 1.86 |
| Industrial Radiographer | 5.28 |
| Nuclear Fuel Processor | 3.38 |
| Reactor Operator | 2.62 |
| Reactor Mechanical Maintainer | 3.47 |
| Uranium Miner Gamma | 1.79 |
| Radon | 1.03 WLM |

* Average of doses ≥0.2 mSv and 0.2 WLM

Average doses received by all workers in an industry are one indicator of how well the industry is controlling occupational dose, but how is the dose distributed? Are there a large number of workers receiving low doses and another large group receiving high doses?

The distribution of the total doses received in the five-year period from 1986 to 1990 for all occupationally exposed workers at all Canadian nuclear power stations is

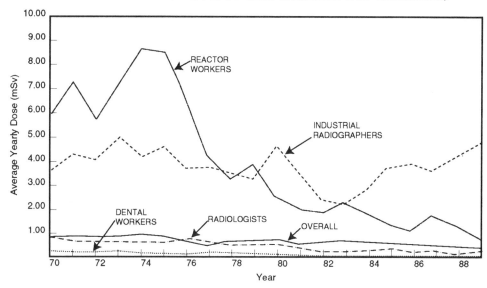

FIGURE 9.2
AVERAGE WHOLE BODY DOSE BY YEAR (SELECTED JOB CATEGORIES)

FIGURE 9.3
CANADIAN NUCLEAR POWER STATION WORKERS
FIVE YEAR DOSE DISTRIBUTION; 1986 – 1990

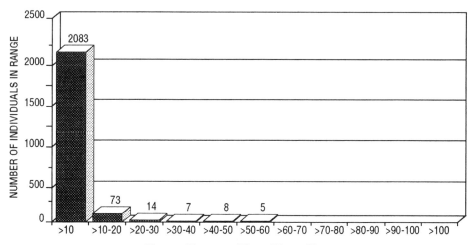

shown in Figure 9.3. The average annual dose for the most highly exposed group of workers in that five-year period did not exceed 12 mSv.

## URANIUM MINING

Uranium mining has been carried out in Canada since the 1930s. Initially the interest was in the medically useful radium that the uranium ore contained, but since the second world war, radium has been replaced in cancer treatment by man-made radionuclides, so that the interest today is in the uranium itself.

Miners are exposed to gamma radiation from the ore, and to radon decay products in the mine atmosphere. In the early days of uranium mining a unit was established for measuring exposure to radon decay products in air. This was called a *Working Level* and initially the guideline for a year's exposure to this airborne workplace contaminant was 12 *Working Level Months* (WLM). This could be received as six months exposure to 2 Working Levels, or four months exposure to 3 Working Levels, etc. As knowledge about the long term health effects of radon decay products increased, the annual exposure value decreased to its current level of 4 WLM, which is the present legal limit.

One WLM is now defined as exposure for 170 hours to a Working Level and is considered equivalent to an external gamma dose to the whole body of about 5 mSv. A Working Level is defined as the quantity of radon decay products in one litre of air which will result in the emission of $1.6 \times 10^{-13}$ joules ($1.3 \times 10^5$ Mev) of alpha radiation energy. The exposure of miners to gamma radiation and to radon decay products has been relatively constant over the past ten-year period.

## AVERAGE ANNUAL DOSES IN NON-URANIUM MINING

Apart from uranium mining, mining is not generally considered radiation work, so other miners are not required to wear dosimeters in Canada. As a result there is not much information on the radiation dose received by Canadian miners, but some is available for non-uranium miners in the United Kingdom from the National Radiological Protection Board in that country. Most coal mines in the U.K. are well ventilated with the result that coal miners there are exposed to relatively low concentrations of radon decay products. Their average annual dose from both radon and external gamma radiation is estimated at 0.6 mSv. In tin and fluorspar mines the radon concentration is considerably higher and the average dose in that type of mining is about 7 mSv. This is much higher than the dose received by the average nuclear station worker or medical x-ray technologist in Canada.

## OCCUPATIONAL DOSE OF AIRLINE CREWS

Passengers and crew of aircraft flying at high altitudes are exposed to high levels of cosmic radiation. On a flight from Montreal to Fredericton the additional dose amounts to about 0.0005 mSv, and the maximum dose rate is about 20 times that on the ground in Montreal. In the United States in 1980 the average annual dose received by about 70,000 crew members of subsonic passenger jets, which fly at about 8 km altitude, was estimated to be between 1 and 2 mSv. The collective dose to this working population is therefore about 100 person·Sv. No Canadian data is available, but the individual doses for Canadian aircrews should be similar to that for their U.S. counterparts. The number of personnel involved is much smaller, so that based on population ratios the collective dose should be approximately ten times less than that for the U.S., about 10 person·Sv. Data from the 1988 report of UNSCEAR suggest somewhat lower doses; the dose to aircrew who fly 600 hours per year at 8 km is given as 1 mSv.

Data from the U.K. is consistent with that from the U.S. Individual doses measured there by the NRPB give an annual dose for aircrew members of about 2 mSv for subsonic passenger flights, and a collective dose of 40 person·Sv. Higher annual average individual doses are received by the crews of the supersonic Concorde.

This is because Concorde flies at a considerably higher altitude than subsonic aircraft and the cosmic dose rate is much higher. The average annual dose to Concorde aircrew is about 2.5 mSv, with up to 15 mSv maximum. Cosmic dose rate is very dependant on solar flares. During solar flares, cosmic radiation doses at the height flown by Concorde on a transatlantic run (19 km) can increase by 10,000 times. Detectors have been provided on Concorde to warn pilots when the dose rate exceeds 0.5 mSv/h, so that they may reduce altitude to take advantage of the shielding provided by the atmosphere.

## DOSES TO ASTRONAUTS

Cosmic radiation is also a source of occupational exposure to astronauts, especially when engaged in activities outside their spacecraft. Information summarized by UNSCEAR in 1988 indicates that for U.S. astronauts the dose per mission is

| SOME ANNUAL OCCUPATIONAL DOSES FROM NATURAL SOURCES | | |
|---|---|---|
| | Average Individual Dose (mSv) | Population Dose (Person·Sv) |
| Aircraft Crew (U.S.A. 1980) | 1 – 2 | 100 |
| Aircraft Crew (U.K. 1987) | 2 (Subsonic) 2.5 (Supersonic) | 40 - |
| Coal Mines (U.K. 1987) | 1.2 | 96 |
| Other Mines (U.K. 1987) | 14 | 28 |
| Uranium Mines (Canada 1991) | 4.5 | 9 |

in the range 0.5 to 5 mSv. On some of the prolonged flights by former Soviet Union astronauts, for example expedition IV on Salut-6 which lasted 175 days, the dose received was 55 mSv. Radiation exposure may be a factor which will limit prolonged space travel.

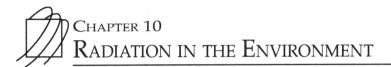

# CHAPTER 10
# RADIATION IN THE ENVIRONMENT

As well as the radioactivity which occurs naturally in the environment, radioactivity is present because of human activities. This includes the widespread use of radionuclides in medicine and industry, but also includes fallout from atmospheric testing of nuclear weapons, leakage from underground nuclear explosions, accidental and routine releases from nuclear facilities and the management of radioactive waste. Whatever the origin, environmental radioactivity leads to human exposure by one or more of several pathways (Figure 10.1) including external irradiation from radionuclides in the air and deposited on the ground, and internal irradiation from the inhalation of airborne radionuclides and their ingestion in food or water.

When radionuclides enter soil or water at a steady rate over long enough periods, a state will eventually be reached when the rate they enter equals the rate at which they leave either by decay or by being transferred elsewhere. The concentrations thereafter remain constant and this condition is known as a 'steady state'.

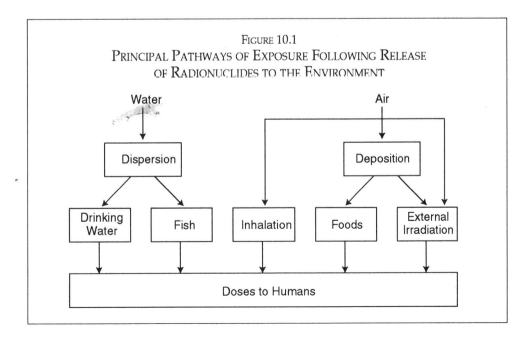

FIGURE 10.1
PRINCIPAL PATHWAYS OF EXPOSURE FOLLOWING RELEASE
OF RADIONUCLIDES TO THE ENVIRONMENT

Because the concentration remains unchanged, the dose rate is also unchanging. It is then convenient to express that rate in terms of an annual dose as was done for natural sources in Chapter 6.

However, many releases are not like this but occur as single short bursts. In such situations, concentrations in affected environmental materials change in time and so do the resulting dose rates. At first, after a single short release to the environment, there is a rise to a peak concentration followed by a decline until the concentration eventually returns to its original level. The rate at which the decline occurs depends on the radionuclides released and their behaviour in the environment. An annual dose cannot be quoted because the value changes from year to year. For this kind of source a better measure of its impact is obtained by summing the doses for each year, from the time radioactivity first appears in the environment to the time when it disappears. The sum is called the 'dose commitment' because once a radionuclide enters the environment, people and sometimes succeeding generations are committed to receiving dose. Dose commitment is used by the United Nations Scientific Committee on the Effects of Atomic Radiation to describe the impacts of various nuclear practices.

# FALLOUT FROM NUCLEAR WEAPONS TESTS

Atmospheric testing of nuclear weapons injected radioactive material into the stratosphere from which it was slowly transferred into the lower atmosphere or troposphere. Most of this test debris was injected between 1950 and 1963, when the Limited Nuclear Test Ban Treaty went into effect. Since then only a few small-scale tests have been carried out.

Most of this radioactive material that went into the atmosphere has now been deposited. Many different radionuclides are formed in a nuclear explosion but most decay rapidly, so that after an initial short period during which they contribute external radiation, they do not present a hazard to people or living things. In the long term, only three, carbon-14, strontium-90 and cesium-137 give significant doses and these do so internally through dietary pathways. Most of the doses to be expected from strontium-90 and cesium-137 have already been delivered, leaving only carbon-14 as the primary source of ongoing radiation dose. The current average dose from weapons testing is about 0.005 mSv a year, about one thirtieth of the corresponding rate in 1963.

According to UNSCEAR the dose commitment per person from past tests of nuclear weapons in the atmosphere for the north temperate zone is 4.5 mSv. This dose commitment is the average for the latitudes from 20° North to 60° North and will be the approximate lifetime dose received by persons living within these latitudes in Canada over the next several hundred years. However, further north the lichen→ caribou → human food chain results in somewhat higher doses.

## CHERNOBYL NUCLEAR ACCIDENT

On April 26, 1986, a power surge in a reactor at the Chernobyl nuclear power station in Ukraine caused an explosion and fire that led to large quantities of radionuclides being released to the atmosphere over the following ten days. The most serious effects were felt locally and in eastern Europe. The population within a 30 km radius of the plant was evacuated, some 90,000 people. This area is contaminated with fission products from the reactor and is still not considered suitable for normal human habitation.

Air currents carried the cloud in both easterly and westerly directions, reaching Canada's east coast on May 6 and west coast on May 7. Radioactive material was detected in rain at Ottawa on May 7 and in air on May 8. The principal radionuclides in the cloud that eventually spread across Canada were iodine-131, cesium-137, cesium-134 and ruthenium-103, but only cesium-137 and iodine-131 made significant contributions to doses. The highest air concentrations occurred on May 10 and by the end of June the activity levels had returned to normal. For the two months of May and June, Health Canada estimated a total dose of 0.00028 mSv per person of which about half was due to external radiation from deposited radionuclides. This dose is much smaller than that from natural background and the corresponding doses from the same incident reported from Japan, the U.S.A. and many countries of Europe.

## RELEASES OF RADIONUCLIDES TO THE ENVIRONMENT

Radionuclides released to the environment come from a wide range of sources, including the nuclear fuel cycle, military establishments, research organizations, hospitals and non-nuclear industries. Release limits for nuclear facilities must be authorized by appropriate federal and provincial authorities. Compliance with authorizations is checked by monitoring effluents and, if appropriate, other environmental materials.

Most of the anthropogenic radioactivity currently entering the environment is from the nuclear power industry. Air, soil water and vegetables around Canadian nuclear generating stations are monitored by the electrical utility, by Health Canada and by provincial authorities.

The nuclear power industry may be conveniently divided into operations or stages, beginning with mining of uranium ore and ending with the final disposal of the spent fuel and other radioactive wastes in an appropriate repository (Figure 10.2).

FIGURE 10.2
NUCLEAR FUEL PRODUCTION AND
USE/WASTE MANAGEMENT

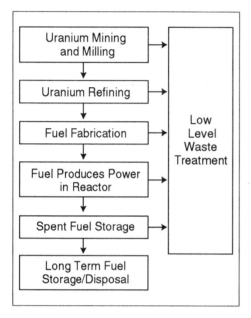

Each stage of the fuel cycle produces its own characteristic type of release. Mining and milling wastes contain mostly uranium, thorium and radium isotopes in powdered rock, slurried in water. The 'tailings' piles created become sources of airborne radon and thoron and their solid decay products, as described in Chapter 6. Refineries and fuel fabrication plants discharge mainly uranium and thorium isotopes. Nuclear reactors discharge radioisotopes of noble gases, tritium and carbon-14 to the atmosphere, and cesium-134, cesium-137 and cobalt-60 to water. The current practice of retaining complete spent fuel bundles either submerged in water storage bays or dry in concrete silos (Figure 13.2), discharges very little radioactivity because of the multiple containment barriers provided. No spent fuel is disposed of in Canada or in any other western country. Much research is underway here and elsewhere to find suitable methods for permanently disposing of spent fuel. A few decades will probably elapse before a safe methodology has been satisfactorily demonstrated.

In most countries other than Canada, a fuel enrichment stage comes before the production of fuel elements, to increase the concentration of uranium-235 above that of natural uranium. Uranium-235 is the isotope of uranium that fissions readily; (see Chapter 11). The CANDU system does not need this enrichment stage.

Also in some of those countries, the fuel after it is removed from the reactor is processed chemically so that unused uranium-235 and plutonium produced in the fuel can be recycled. This step to recover the fissile plutonium may be useful sometime in the future but is not necessary in the CANDU system at this time. Fuel leaving a CANDU reactor contains less uranium-235 per kilogram of total uranium than is thrown away in the waste stream of a typical reprocessing plant.

## Waste Disposal and Waste Management

Nuclear power produces most but not all the radioactive waste in Canada. Some comes from laboratories processing radionuclides for medicine, industry and research, where their use generates further waste. Waste management operations are designed to safeguard the public and to minimize doses received by workers. Different techniques are applied depending on the activity level, the concentration, the strength of associated external radiation fields and on how long it will take before the radioactivity decays to insignificance.

Safety is achieved by isolating the waste from people; by remoteness which reduces the chance of people gaining access to it; and by immobilizing it so that it is less likely to escape and reach people.

Spent fuel is hazardous but is in some ways the easiest to manage. It contains high levels of radioactivity at high concentrations, some of which will take several millions of years to decay away. In the Canadian system the radionuclides are already immobile, locked inside the crystal structure of the ceramic uranium oxide fuel which is itself inside at least two metal cans. Achieving isolation then is the main problem to be addressed and Canada, like other countries, is looking at incarcerating the spent fuel deep (up to 1 km) inside bedrock.

Most of the rest of the radioactive waste that arises from nuclear power and elsewhere is less hazardous. The amounts are smaller and the concentrations lower, with radioactive half lives of hundreds, not millions of years. Some of it, in smoke detectors for example, is so small in amount it can be disposed of as if it were non-radioactive. Most radioactivity incorporated in consumer products may be disposed of in this way. High level gaseous and liquid wastes are solidified and the volume of solid wastes reduced. Solidification alone helps immobilize the radionuclides, but encapsulating them in bitumen, concrete or glass adds still more protection. After that they are buried. Some, those with a long half-life, may be placed in rock cavities or may be buried in deep soil, but above the water table. A concrete cover is required to keep out water and prevent inadvertent and premature exposure or disturbance by drillers and diggers.

Nuclear generating stations also produce large volumes of waste which is low in total activity, short-lived and of low concentrations. Spills of lightly contaminated water must be mopped up, creating paper or cloth wastes. Pipes, valves and other parts of radioactive systems have to be replaced. The equipment removed must be treated as radioactive waste. As the waste is low in concentration but large in total bulk, it is either incinerated if this is possible, or placed in concrete trenches or shallow, land burial trenches on controlled property with restricted public access. Where this method has been adopted there is no evidence that it has ever resulted in doses to the public of more than a minute fraction of background. Nevertheless, improvements in ways to handle this waste are still being sought.

Finally, there are gaseous and liquid wastes too large in bulk and containing radioactivity too low in concentration to be treated successfully at reasonable cost. These are released to the atmosphere and water. Typically the wastes contain inert gases (called 'inert', because they do not react chemically and are absorbed very poorly), tritium in water vapour, and carbon-14. The amounts that can be released this way are carefully controlled. The Atomic Energy Control Board regulates the releases so that the doses received by the most exposed members of the public do not exceed a very small fraction of the annual dose limit. Impacts of these small releases were discussed in an earlier section.

## NON-NUCLEAR SOURCES

Human activities that use soil or rock as source material may increase the local concentrations of primordial radionuclides and their decay products even though, unlike uranium mining, they are not intended for nuclear processes. For example, simply moving materials from a place where their concentration is naturally high to another place where it is normally low will increase radiation exposure at the receiving site. When soil or rock is treated physically or chemically, concentrations of radionuclides may coincidentally increase either in the product itself or in the waste stream. For example, concentrations of uranium and thorium and their decay products are usually lower in coal than in soils, but when coal is burned, concentrations of these radionuclides in the remaining ash is increased about seven or eight times what they were in the unburned coal. Concentrations in the waste are then higher than in the native soils. A small fraction of ash escapes to the air but the rest is disposed in landfill sites. At the boundary of the Nanticoke Thermal Generating Station in Ontario, one of the largest coal-burning generating stations in the world, the committed dose from ingestion following the fallout of airborne fly-ash on vegetation at the boundary fence, is estimated to be 0.00027 mSv per year of operation. This is about 1% of the corresponding dose at the site boundary of the nuclear generating station at Pickering in Ontario.

Several other human activities either concentrate naturally occurring radionuclides or increase human exposure to naturally occurring ionizing radiation. The increased radiation dose received by airline crews, especially Concorde crews, has been discussed previously. Phosphate rock contains relatively high concentrations of primordial radionuclides. Treating it to produce fertilizer increases the radionuclide concentrations in the product rather than in the waste. Nevertheless, at least some of the waste still has relatively high concentrations of primordial radionuclides and this has to be considered when disposing of it. In Japan, the phosphogypsum produced from the waste of wet fertilizer plants is used to produce wallboard. According to UNSCEAR, use of this wallboard in buildings increases the annual dose rate inside by about 0.5 mSv per year. Other industrial activities, such as the use of Zircon sand (a sand containing the element zirconium) for refractories, and various non-uranium metal mining and processing, result in small additional doses to workers and the public. This is due to the presence of small amounts of uranium-238 and thorium-232 in the raw materials and waste streams.

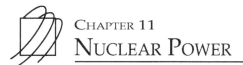

CHAPTER 11

# NUCLEAR POWER

In the late 1930s, scientists in Germany discovered that the atoms of uranium, a naturally occurring radioactive material, not only disintegrated by emitting beta radiation but would occasionally split, or fission, into two approximately equal parts. In this fissioning process energy is released. (Figure 11.1)

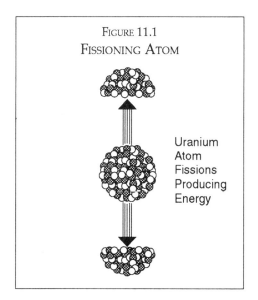

FIGURE 11.1
FISSIONING ATOM

Uranium
Atom
Fissions
Producing
Energy

The energy production can be determined by the famous relationship established by Einstein.

$$E = mc^2$$

This relationship says that if mass can be converted into energy by some process then the amount of energy E obtained in units called ergs is obtained by multiplying the mass in grams by the velocity of light (in cm/sec) squared.

In fission, mass is converted into energy. If the mass (or weight) of a uranium atom before fissioning is compared with the mass of the parts afterwards, then there is a loss of mass. The difference has been converted into energy.

Mass Before = Mass After + Energy

One gram of mass converted into energy produces:

$9 \times 10^{20}$ ergs, or

$9 \times 10^{13}$ joules, or

$2.5 \times 10^7$ kilowatt-hours

This amount of energy would keep an electric kettle boiling for over 1,000 years (if it did not run out of water).

One of the discoveries essential to the further development of nuclear energy, both for military and peaceful purposes, was that during fission one or two neutrons are emitted at high speed, and if one of these neutrons hits another uranium nucleus it may cause that nucleus to fission. The production of energy by this process was now practical. If one fission could produce another fission then a series, or chain, of reactions could be started. If more than one fission is produced by each fission then the number of reactions in the reaction chain will increase. The process may be likened to dominoes being lined up so that the first on the line to fall causes its neighbour to fall and so on, (Figure 11.2). This is a steady chain reaction.

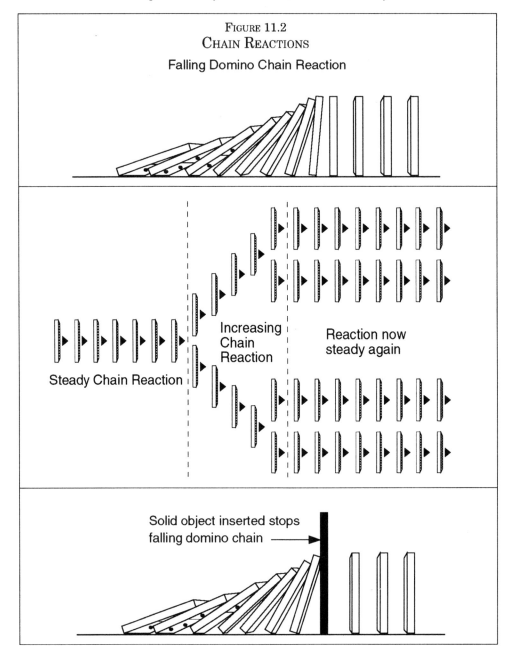

FIGURE 11.2
CHAIN REACTIONS
Falling Domino Chain Reaction

Steady Chain Reaction

Increasing Chain Reaction

Reaction now steady again

Solid object inserted stops falling domino chain

If one domino causes two to fall, as in the second diagram, then the reaction will increase. If, on the other hand solid rods are inserted into a line of dominoes that line will stop falling. This is similar to a neutron chain reaction and how such a reaction may be increased or decreased.

Further discoveries were that if neutrons were slowed down after being emitted during fission they were more likely to fission another uranium atom, and that uranium-235 was very much more likely to fission than the other main isotope of uranium, uranium-238. The important essential facts for the design of a controlled chain reaction were now in place.

•   uranium had to be assembled in an array, to give the neutrons produced when a nucleus fissions the opportunity to hit another uranium atom;

•   neutrons emitted from fissions had to be slowed down, or moderated in speed without being absorbed;

•   a material which absorbs neutrons had to be capable of being inserted into the assembly to control or stop the reaction.

There are only a few substances that may be used to slow down or moderate the speed of neutrons without absorbing too many of them.   These *moderators* are graphite (a form of carbon), water and *heavy water*.   An assembly of graphite with natural uranium, or heavy water with natural uranium, can sustain a chain reaction.   Ordinary water absorbs neutrons quite readily, so to sustain a chain reaction with it as a moderator the uranium has to be enriched in the uranium-235 isotope.

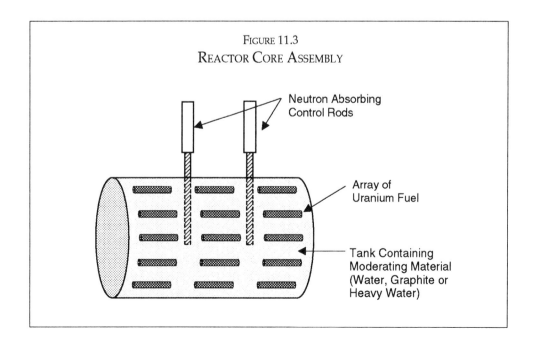

FIGURE 11.3
REACTOR CORE ASSEMBLY

Neutron Absorbing
Control Rods

Array of
Uranium Fuel

Tank Containing
Moderating Material
(Water, Graphite or
Heavy Water)

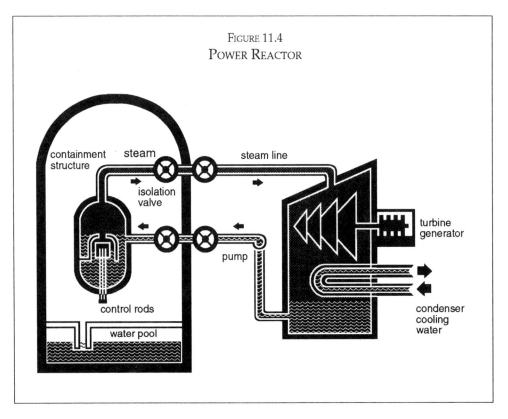

FIGURE 11.4
POWER REACTOR

The device used to initiate, contain and control fission is called a *nuclear reactor*. A practical reactor consists of a tank containing a matrix of uranium fuel, surrounded by one of the moderating materials and with provision for insertion of a neutron absorber into the array, (Figure 11.3).

The various nuclear power stations which have been developed in the world employ a reactor which is an assembly of uranium fuel, a moderator and a system to remove heat. The heat produces steam, usually in a boiler, which drives a turbine which turns a generator to produce electricity, (Figure 11.4).

Countries have developed reactors with different combinations of materials for fuel, moderator and heat removal as shown in the table on the next page. The reason why different countries took different paths in reactor development is related to their involvement with nuclear weapons and submarines. Uranium highly enriched in the isotope U-235 is needed for a nuclear weapon.

Both the United States and the former Soviet Union had built the costly facilities needed to enrich uranium in the U-235 isotope, and water is of course a low cost moderator, so both these countries developed reactors using these materials. Neither Canada nor the United Kingdom had enrichment facilities and so have not

| Reactor Type | Fuel | Moderator | Heat Transport |
|---|---|---|---|
| US PWR | Enriched $UO_2$ | Water | Water |
| US BWR | Enriched $UO_2$ | Water | Water |
| USSR PWR | Enriched $UO_2$ | Water | Water |
| USSR RBMK | Enriched $UO_2$ | Graphite | Water |
| UK Gas/Graphite | Natural U | Graphite | Carbon Dioxide |
| UK AGR | Natural $UO_2$ | Graphite | Helium |
| CANDU | Natural $UO_2$ | Heavy Water | Heavy Water |

PWR – Pressurized Water Reactor
BWR – Boiling Water Reactor
AGR – Advanced Gas Reactor
RBMK – Russian for Water Cooled
Reactor Moderated by
Graphite (Chernobyl Type)

developed power reactors using enriched uranium. As part of the combined allied efforts in the second world war, Canada had been producing heavy water, so this, which has proven to be the best of all moderators, was available to develop reactors in Canada. The result was the type known as CANDU, (CANadian Deuterium Uranium.)

## THE CANDU REACTOR

The first CANDU reactor, NPD, was built by AECL at Rolphton, Ontario, and produced its first power in 1962. It was operated by Ontario Hydro. The first full-scale CANDU reactor was the Douglas Point reactor situated on Lake Huron. This was also built by AECL and

operated by Ontario Hydro. First power was produced in 1967. There are now twenty reactors in five large nuclear power stations in operation in Ontario. Single reactor nuclear power stations are also in service in the provinces of New Brunswick and Quebec, (Figure 11.5).

Both Ontario Hydro and AECL have continued to develop power reactors. The reactors they have developed differ in detail but are similar in principle to the early reactor units. A typical CANDU design is shown, (Figure 11.6). The fuel is in bundles (Figure 11.7) in pressure tubes which pass through a large tank called a calandria, containing heavy water to moderate the neutrons produced in the fissioning process occurring in the fuel bundles.

Control rods which absorb neutrons penetrate into the calandria between the pressure tubes. Heavy water passes over the fuel bundles transferring the heat produced in them to a boiler where ordinary (or light) water is boiled to produce

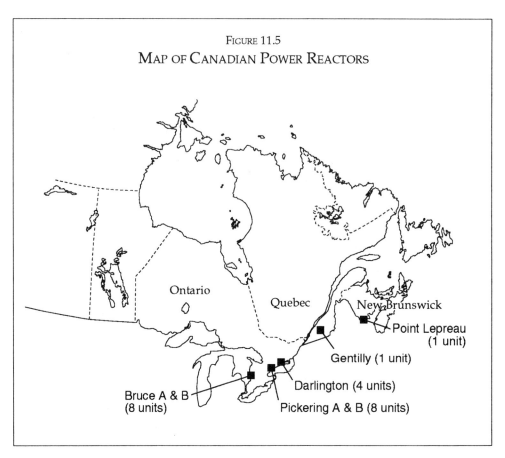

FIGURE 11.5
MAP OF CANADIAN POWER REACTORS

Ontario

Quebec

New Brunswick

Point Lepreau
(1 unit)

Gentilly (1 unit)

Darlington (4 units)

Bruce A & B
(8 units)

Pickering A & B (8 units)

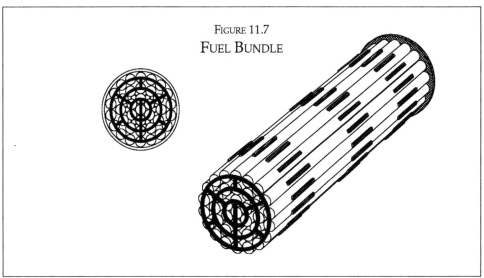

FIGURE 11.7
FUEL BUNDLE

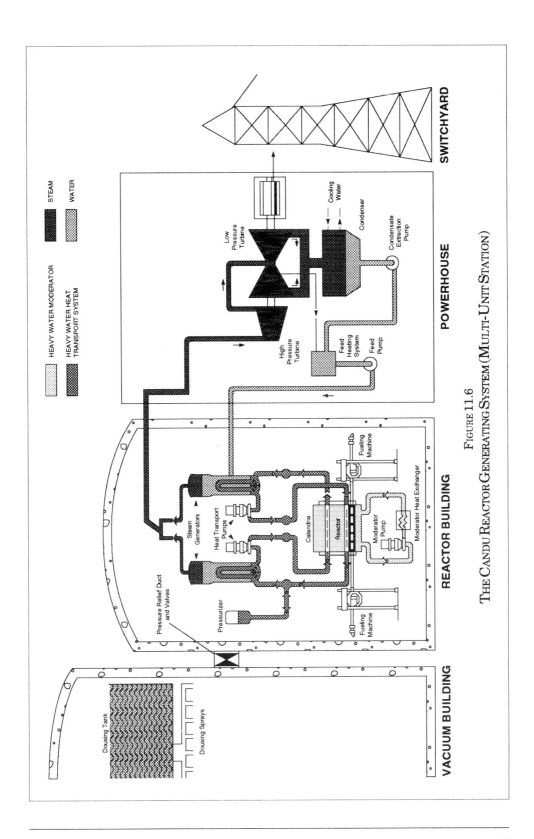

FIGURE 11.6

THE CANDU REACTOR GENERATING SYSTEM (MULTI-UNIT STATION)

steam which drives the turbine. The fuel material is uranium dioxide ($UO_2$), a ceramic-like material which is very stable and does not burn. When the reactor operates, the U-235 in the fuel is consumed and eventually has to be replaced. The spent fuel contains fission products which are highly radioactive.

Fuelling machines are designed to attach to each end of a pressure tube, remove a plug closing the end of the tube and push old fuel into one machine and new fuel from the other into the reactor. The spent fuel is transferred from the fuelling machines to a spent fuel bay. This is a structure almost identical to a large, deep swimming pool. The spent fuel bundles can be safely stored there for as long as is necessary to come to a decision about their eventual disposition. The fuel bundles, at some time in the future, could be a useful source of new fuel material as each bundle contains plutonium-239 which will fission like uranium-235. Discovery of large deposits of very high grade uranium in Canada and Australia make it unlikely that use will be made of this fuel for a long time, if ever.

In a reactor not all the uranium fissions. Typically in a CANDU reactor each kilogram of uranium produces $3.5 \times 10^4$ kilowatt-hours of energy. About 70,000 kg of coal would have to be burned to produce the same amount of energy. Therein lies an advantage of nuclear power – the mass of fuel and spent fuel is comparatively small. There are also no combustion gases to produce acid rain or increase the greenhouse effect. The disadvantages include safety concerns. Reactors have the ability to go to very high power levels very quickly, and after operating for some time contain large quantities of hazardous radioactive materials which must be managed painstakingly.

## REACTOR SAFETY

In a reactor the fission process is the eventual source of heat. Although each fission only produces a small amount of energy (heat), the number of fissions occurring per second in a power reactor is a huge number. Each fission produces two fission product atoms, (Figure 11.8).

Fission products are usually radioactive, so that as a reactor operates, there is an accumulation of radioactive fission products in the fuel bundles.

Eventually the fissionable uranium-235 in the reactor becomes used up, and if not replaced by new fuel, the nuclear chain reaction would stop. At the time a fuel bundle has most of its fissionable uranium-235 used up, a large quantity of fission products have accumulated in the bundle. The fuel bundle is highly radioactive and has to be transferred from the reactor by remote handling mechanisms and stored under at least three metres of water in the spent fuel bay. There are about 4,000 fuel bundles in the reactor, so within it there is an enormous inventory of radioactive fission products. It is important that these fission products do not escape to the environment. They must be retained within the heat transport system or station buildings, and the reactor power must be strictly controlled. The technology or engineering to achieve this is known as *Reactor Safety*.

There are two characteristics of a power reactor that are important to the objective of keeping fission products within fuel bundles. The first is that a reactor can very quickly go from low power to very high power. If not controlled it could reach power levels that could destroy the fuel bundles, the structure of the reactor and even the buildings containing the reactor structure. Referring back to the domino comparison, the rate at which power rises is the equivalent of a change in a short time from a few dominoes falling per second to millions per second. An objective of reactor safety is to prevent any such uncontrolled power increases.

The second characteristic important to safety is that fission products which accumulate in fuel bundles produce energy when their radioactive disintegration occurs. This fission product energy continues to be produced even after the reactor is shut down. Initially, just after a reactor is shut down, this fission product energy is about 7% of the full power energy. The energy is enough to melt the fuel bundles (and so let fission products escape) if cooling is not maintained. Therefore a second objective of reactor safety is to maintain fuel cooling at all times.

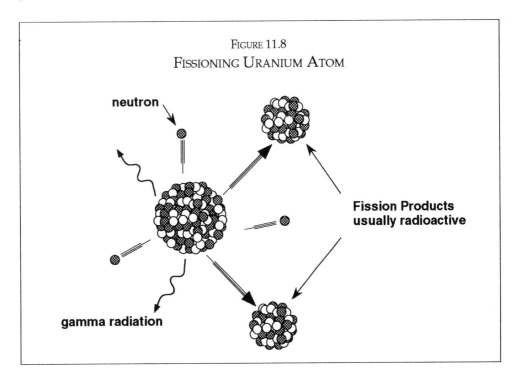

FIGURE 11.8
FISSIONING URANIUM ATOM

neutron

Fission Products
usually radioactive

gamma radiation

If the precautions taken to control the reactor and keep cooling the fuel fail, then additional measures are taken to ensure that radioactive material does not harm any member of the public. The two most important of these measures are to contain the reactor system within a low leakage building (the containment system), and to require that no homes are built within a radius of at least a kilometre of a power reactor.

## CONTROLLING REACTOR POWER IN NORMAL OPERATION

Prevention of the release of radioactive material is achieved by a combination of high quality design, operating procedures and training of station staff. In normal operation, control of the reactor is done by the *Regulating System.* This system controls the power level and only permits it to change slowly. The system is of high quality and is usually triplicated. Each of the triplicated systems can be taken out of service for testing and maintenance while the reactor is operating.

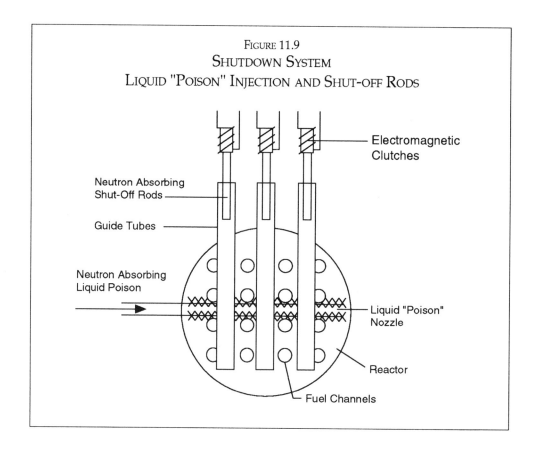

FIGURE 11.9
SHUTDOWN SYSTEM
LIQUID "POISON" INJECTION AND SHUT-OFF RODS

Electromagnetic Clutches

Neutron Absorbing Shut-Off Rods

Guide Tubes

Neutron Absorbing Liquid Poison

Liquid "Poison" Nozzle

Reactor

Fuel Channels

## SPECIAL SAFETY SYSTEMS

Quite separate from, and independent of, the Regulating System are systems called *Special Safety Systems.* These systems are designed to make it highly unlikely that radioactive material will be released in any circumstances.

The first of the Special Safety Systems is the shutdown system. A modern CANDU reactor has two shutdown systems, (Figure 11.9). These are independent of each other and are each capable of shutting down the reactor. One of these consists of neutron absorbers that are poised ready to be inserted into the reactor to stop the chain reaction; (in the domino comparison it is like inserting solid pieces of metal into the lines of falling dominoes). A second system employed is one that is poised ready to inject a liquid neutron absorber or "poison" such as boron, into the heavy water moderator of the reactor. The systems can be tested and maintained without affecting their ability to ensure that they will always operate when required to shut down the reactor.

## EMERGENCY COOLING SYSTEMS

In addition to the normal systems that are available to keep the fuel bundles cool, the reactor has systems to provide cooling in an emergency. The emergency injection system is designed to inject cooling water at high pressure onto the fuel bundles if there is a break in the heat transport system and normal cooling is lost.

## CONTAINMENT SYSTEMS

Most power reactors are housed in buildings designed to contain the steam pressure and the radioactive fission products if a break occurs in the high pressure heat transport system. Exceptions to this are some of the British gas reactors and the former Soviet RBMK reactors. U.S. power reactors are contained in a building that is designed to withstand the full pressure rise that occurs if a break occurs in the system. In the CANDU design, containment is of two types. In the 600-megawatt (electrical) AECL single reactor models, any steam released by a heat transport system break is cooled by a cold water spray system (the dousing system). The resulting rise in pressure is contained in the reactor building with very low leakage to the environment. Ontario Hydro reactors in their multi-unit stations have a unique containment design, (Figure 11.10). Each of the reactor buildings is connected to a large-volume building by a duct and pressure relief valves. The air in this building is maintained well below normal atmospheric pressure and so it is known as a vacuum building.

A rise in pressure caused by steam from a break in the heat transport system causes the valves in the duct to open and connects the reactor building to the low pressure in the vacuum building. The steam entering the vacuum building is sprayed and condensed by cold water from a dousing tank. The final pressure in both buildings is less than atmospheric, keeping any release of radioactive materials to low levels.

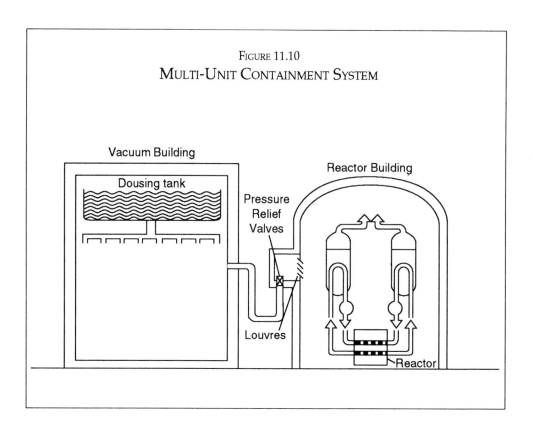

FIGURE 11.10
MULTI-UNIT CONTAINMENT SYSTEM

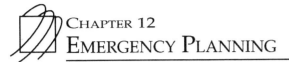

CHAPTER 12
# EMERGENCY PLANNING

## PURPOSE OF EMERGENCY PLANNING

Nuclear reactors, especially power reactors, possess the potential for accidents with serious consequences. The likelihood of such an accident occurring at a Canadian power reactor is low but it is prudent to carry out emergency planning for the protection of the public and station personnel. Some notable reactor accidents include those at the NRX reactor at Chalk River Ontario in 1952, the Windscale reactor in the United Kingdom in 1956, the Three Mile Island reactor in the U.S.A. in 1979, and the Chernobyl reactor in the former Soviet Union in 1986. Analyses of these and other reactor accidents have resulted in improved reactor safety and provided the basis for emergency planning.

Nuclear reactors have this accident potential for many reasons. If loss of control of the chain reaction occurs, a reactor may produce power at levels much greater than its intended full power level. In addition, if the reactor has been operational at power for any length of time, the fuel bundles in the core contain large quantities of hazardous radioactive fis-

sion products. Finally, the power being produced by a reactor cannot be fully shut off; the fission products that have accumulated in the fuel continue to produce energy. Immediately after a reactor has been shut down from full power this fission product energy is about 7% of the full power level. For a 1,500 megawatt thermal power station this residual heat is about 100 megawatts of thermal energy, which is about the heat energy that could be produced by 100,000 electric kettles. These characteristics of a nuclear reactor require the installation of special safety systems to ensure that accidents will have an extremely low probability. Special safety systems for reactors have been discussed in some detail in Chapter 11. To summarize, they include protective systems to limit reactor power, cooling systems to prevent overheating of the fuel, and systems to contain escaping fission products. They must meet the licensing requirements of the Atomic Energy Control Board. In addition, the Atomic Energy Control Board requires the reactor operator to have satisfactory emergency planning in place. This is regarded as a supplementary level of protection that is never expected to be used, in somewhat the same manner as household fire insurance.

## Responsibility for Emergency Planning

Regulatory responsibility for nuclear emergency planning in Canada is shared. The Atomic Energy Control Board will grant a licence to a utility to operate a power reactor if it is satisfied that the design is safe, that an acceptable on-site emergency plan is in place and that a provincial off-site emergency plan exists. The regulatory responsibility for the off-site plan rests with the province within which the reactor is situated. Since many emergency forces which would be deployed are under municipal control, the municipalities near a plant also prepare emergency plans. However, if an accident causes the release of radioactive material which crosses international or provincial boundaries, then a number of federal agencies in addition to the Atomic Energy Control Board become involved, to deal with such things as international communications and assistance arrangements. The total emergency planning necessary in Canada for a reactor accident must coordinate the plans of all agencies at the various levels of government.

UTILITY PLANS

MUNICIPAL PLANS

PROVINCIAL PLANS

FEDERAL PLANS

If an uncontrolled high power level occurred, if fuel became overheated and if in addition the containment failed, then fission products could be released to the atmosphere. Those that are most likely to be released are either gaseous or volatile. Fission products of importance in these categories are xenon-133 and krypton-88, which are gaseous, the radioactive iodine isotopes, which are volatile, and the radioactive cesiums, which are semi-volatile.

A release, if it occurs, may be a short term or 'puff' release, or it could extend over a period of days, or both. The radioactive cloud or plume emitted may expose people in several ways. Radiation from the radionuclides in the cloud would cause direct external exposure for anyone not shielded from it. This direct exposure would cease as the cloud moved on and was dispersed by the prevailing wind. Exposure may also result from inhalation of radionuclides in the plume. If the release contained only noble gases then no further radiation doses would be received after the passage of the plume. If the plume contained radioiodine or the semi-volatile cesium fission products, then, besides the dose that would be received directly from the plume and by inhalation, a dose would be received from radioactive material deposited on the ground surface and from ingestion of contaminated vegetables and cereals. These foods may have radioactive contamination deposited on their surfaces, or may have absorbed radioactivity from contaminated soil. Milk from dairy cattle raised on pasture contaminated with

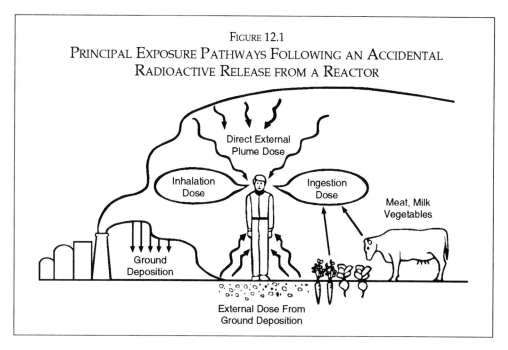

FIGURE 12.1
PRINCIPAL EXPOSURE PATHWAYS FOLLOWING AN ACCIDENTAL
RADIOACTIVE RELEASE FROM A REACTOR

Direct External
Plume Dose

Inhalation
Dose

Ingestion
Dose

Meat, Milk
Vegetables

Ground
Deposition

External Dose From
Ground Deposition

iodine-131 will be contaminated. Meat from livestock raised on pasture contaminated with fission product cesium may be contaminated. Emergency planning must consider all these possible exposure routes and develop actions which will minimize potentially harmful public exposure.

## ON-SITE EMERGENCY PLANNING

Each nuclear power station in Canada has an on-site emergency plan as required by the Atomic Energy Control Board. Actions under the plan include establishing control of potential releases, protection of the station staff, evaluation of the possible extent of the emergency and notification of provincial authorities responsible for off-site emergency actions. The station staff will carry out initial off-site radiation surveys and contamination measurements and, if conditions warrant it, they will request local authorities such as the police to take actions necessary to protect the public.

## OFF-SITE EMERGENCY PLANNING

Off-site emergency plans for nuclear stations are the responsibility of the province. Plans for stations are similar, but not identical, from province to province. Planning is usually based on the emergency having three phases:

- the plume exposure phase – this is usually of short duration when a radioactive gas cloud is being released from the station;

- the ingestion phase – this phase occurs generally after the plume has passed and radioactivity has been deposited on the ground and may enter food chains;

- the recovery phase – this phase follows the ingestion phase and is when actions are being taken to restore conditions in affected areas to normal. This phase could be prolonged.

Emergency actions under the plan are directed by a provincial executive group, or director, supported by an operations group, a technical group and an information group. On instruction by the executive group, the operations group directs off-site forces such as the provincial police, or requests municipal officials to direct their forces. The technical group provides advice on radiological conditions and projected conditions and actions to be taken to minimize dose to the public. The information group assembles data from all groups involved in the emergency. This enables prompt release of consistent and accurate reports of the situation to the public by provincial government, municipal and utility spokespersons.

Certain protective measures are preplanned. This is done for access control, evacuation and sheltering, and restrictions on water and food.

| PLANNED PROTECTIVE MEASURES IN AN EMERGENCY |
| --- |
| Sheltering Indoors |
| Distribution of Iodine Tablets |
| Temporary Evacuation |
| Consumption Ban on Contaminated Foods |

Milk and other dairy products require special consideration because of the exposure pathway for radioiodine from the plume to pasture, to cow, to milk, and finally to people. A person consuming milk contaminated with iodine-131 will receive a large dose to the thyroid because iodine-131 concentrates in that organ. Children are of special concern because of the relatively large role of milk in their diet. A specific protective measure for this exposure pathway is the consumption of stable iodine tablets. These are usually potassium iodide or iodate tablets. The tablets flood the thyroid with stable iodine preventing uptake of the radioactive iodine. To be effective they must be taken immediately before, or within about five hours of, the exposure.

Most off-site provincial plans have established values of dose rate in public areas or levels of radioactivity in food, milk, etc., at which specific protective measures will be implemented. These are known as *Intervention Levels*. Intervention Levels are usually ranges and not single values. This permits some judgment to be made depending on the circumstances of a particular emergency. An important consideration is whether the benefit to be derived from the implementation outweighs any adverse effect associated with the action. All provinces with nuclear power programs have off-site emergency plans. Intervention Levels and other preplanned measures differ significantly from one province to another, so that there is not a common set for Canada. Examples of Intervention Levels are shown in the accompanying table for the province of Ontario.

**EXAMPLES OF PROTECTIVE MEASURES AND INTERVENTION LEVELS FROM THE PROVINCE OF ONTARIO EMERGENCY PLAN**

| Protective Measure | Organ | Lower Intervention Level (mSv) | Upper Intervention Level (mSv) |
|---|---|---|---|
| Sheltering | Whole Body | 1 | 10 |
|  | Thyroid | 3 | 30 |
| Evacuation | Whole Body | 10 | 100 |
|  | Single Organ | 30 | 300 |
| Administration of Stable Iodine | Thyroid | 30 | 300 |
| Food Controls | Whole Body | 0.5 | 5 |
|  |  | 1.5 | 15 |

The federal government is responsible for taking action in nuclear accidents involving two or more provinces, or one occurring in another country, or involving equipment from another country, e.g. a crashed nuclear powered satellite. Federal agencies and departments take action according to the Federal Nuclear Emergency Response Plan (FNERP) for which Health Canada is the lead agency. This department also maintains a radiological monitoring network covering all Canada. The monitoring system can detect airborne contamination arising from major accidents in other countries, such as from the Chernobyl accident. Many federal departments have responsibilities under the FNERP. Emergency Preparedness Canada, Environment Canada and the Atomic Energy Control Board have major roles. The plan was implemented fully in 1988 in preparation for the reentry of the COSMOS 1900 satellite of the former Soviet Union, and was poised but stood down as unnecessary during the Chernobyl event.

Widespread radioactive contamination resulted in Europe from the Chernobyl accident. This has highlighted the need for international agreements for notification of accidents and provisions for assistance. The wide variation in Intervention Levels from country to country in Europe also caused confusion and public loss of confidence in national governments. In 1986, Canada signed an agreement for cooperation with the United States on nuclear emergencies, and in 1990 signed international agreements on notification and the provision of assistance following nuclear incidents.

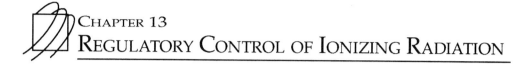

# CHAPTER 13
# REGULATORY CONTROL OF IONIZING RADIATION

## THE LAWS AND THEIR ADMINISTRATION

Laws governing the use of radioactive materials, radiation emitting devices and exposure to ionizing radiation exist in Canada at both federal and provincial government levels. At the federal level the principal legal instruments for this purpose are the:

- RADIATION EMITTING DEVICES ACT and the

- ATOMIC ENERGY CONTROL ACT

The *Radiation Emitting Devices Act* prescribes standards for devices which emit ionizing radiation, to protect the health and safety of Canadians. This act and regulations written under it are administered by Health Canada. The legislation controls radiation emitting equipment such as x-ray machines being imported and sold in Canada.

However, the responsibility for controlling the *use* of radiation emitting devices like dental x-ray machines belongs to the provinces. Provinces regulate and monitor the exposure to ionizing radiation that may result from radiation emitting devices (but not from radioactive materials). Some provinces such as Saskatchewan have prepared their own legislation for the control of exposure to ionizing radiation. This shows that the legislative base for controlling exposure to ionizing radiation is not clear cut. Despite this, the system works surprisingly well.

Among other things, the *Atomic Energy Control Act* and the *Atomic Energy Control Regulations* written under the act, control the use of radioactive materials and fissile materials or processes which could be used in a chain reaction. Protection of the health, safety and security of Canadians is the purpose of the Act.

The Atomic Energy Control Board administers the *Atomic Energy Control Act* and has the leading role in the regulation of nuclear facilities and the use of nuclear materials. Control Board members are appointed by the federal government and are chosen for their competence in appropriate fields such as science, engineering and medicine. The Board itself consists of five members. Four of the five members are appointed directly by the federal government by Order-in-Council.

The fifth is the President of the National Research Council, who is a member by virtue of his or her office. Control Board staff implement the regulatory policies established by the Board.

## REGULATION AND LICENSING OF NUCLEAR FACILITIES AND MATERIALS

Nuclear facilities that are regulated by the Control Board include power and research reactors, uranium mines, mills and refineries, nuclear fuel fabrication plants, particle accelerators, heavy water plants and radioactive waste management facilities.

The licensing process for all nuclear facilities follows the same general pattern. There are three major stages:

- site acceptance,
- construction approval,
- issuance of an operating licence.

At each stage the applicant is required to show that its facility can be built and operated without undue risk to workers, the public and the environment. Throughout the lifespan of the facility the Control Board monitors its performance to ensure that licence conditions are being met. Project officers are attached to nuclear power stations for this purpose.

At the end of the useful life of a facility it must be decommissioned in a way that is acceptable to the Control Board. The site must be restored to unrestricted use, or managed until it no longer presents a hazard to health, safety, security or the environment.

## REGULATION OF NUCLEAR MATERIALS

Nuclear materials are either radionuclides or "prescribed items or substances". Prescribed items or substances are primarily equipment or materials that could be used for the production or application of nuclear energy. This includes, for example, equipment that could be used to separate isotopes, control rods for nuclear reactors and equipment for fabricating nuclear fuel. Canada is committed to the peaceful uses of nuclear energy and the controls are intended to prevent possible misuse of this powerful energy source.

The Control Board issues a large number of radioisotope licenses. A radioisotope license specifies the conditions that must be met by the user. Control Board inspectors check at intervals that these conditions are being met. In 1992, there were about 3,800 licenses in force distributed widely over Canada, (Figure 13.1). These include permits for radioactive sources used in medical diagnosis and treatment of disease (discussed in detail in Chapter 7), and for sources used in industry and research (discussed in detail in Chapter 8).

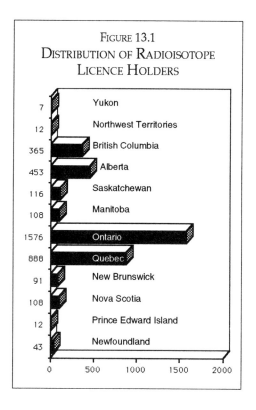

FIGURE 13.1
DISTRIBUTION OF RADIOISOTOPE
LICENCE HOLDERS

| | |
|---|---|
| 7 | Yukon |
| 12 | Northwest Territories |
| 365 | British Columbia |
| 453 | Alberta |
| 116 | Saskatchewan |
| 108 | Manitoba |
| 1576 | Ontario |
| 888 | Quebec |
| 91 | New Brunswick |
| 108 | Nova Scotia |
| 12 | Prince Edward Island |
| 43 | Newfoundland |

0    500   1000   1500   2000

## RADIOACTIVE WASTE MANAGEMENT REGULATION

Nuclear power production, uranium mining and refining, and other nuclear activities produce radioactive wastes. These wastes may vary from spent fuel, which is highly radioactive, to mildly radioactive rags used to clean up a spill of contaminated water. The Control Board regulates the management of radioactive waste to ensure that it causes no hazard to the health or safety of people or to the environment.

Radioactive wastes that have short radioactive half-lives are of minor concern because they lose their radioactivity rapidly. For example technetium-99m, which is widely used in hospitals to diagnose certain illnesses, has a half-life of six hours. This means that in a period of a week any technetium-99m will have decayed to less than four billionths ($4 \times 10^{-9}$) of its original activity.

Some radioactive wastes contain radionuclides which have long half-lives so that such wastes have to be managed to ensure that they will not create problems for future generations. Spent reactor fuel is highly radioactive and contains some very long-lived radionuclides. Currently, spent fuel is either being stored underwater in large pools at reactor sites or inside welded steel containers in concrete "silos" (Figure 13.2). These are safe but interim waste management solutions to be used until a disposal facility, which ensures long term isolation from the biosphere, is completely evaluated and approved by the Control Board.

## TRANSPORTATION OF RADIOACTIVE MATERIALS

The Control Board regulates the packaging, preparation for shipment and receipt of radioactive materials through administration of the *Transportation Packaging of Radioactive Materials Regulations*. As well, the Board co-operates with Transport Canada in regulating the carriage of radioactive materials under the *Transportation of Dangerous Goods Act*.

Shipments of radioactive materials may be made in approved packaging or by

---

special arrangements on a case by case basis. To receive approval, packaging must meet established performance standards, which for shipment of highly radioactive material are very stringent. This type of packaging must withstand a series of tests – heavy impact, fire, and submersion in water. Packages which have been certified in this way in some countries have survived the test of being hit by a locomotive travelling at 165 km per hour.

There are approximately 750,000 packages containing radioactive materials transported each year in Canada. The frequency with which incidents or accidents occur is less than one in 20,000 shipments made, and in only about 10% of these is any radioactive material spilled. Accidents in which significant quantities of radioactive material is spilled are very rare, and to date no personal injuries due to radiation exposure have occurred.

## REGULATORY CONTROL RESULTS

The Control Board monitors the use of radioactive materials and, if necessary, prosecutes licensees who violate regulations or licensing conditions. In the period from April 1, 1991, to March 31, 1992, among some 90,000 monitored workers there were 11 cases in which accumulated radiation doses exceeded the regulatory limits. In the same period 13 prosecutions were initiated. The distribution of the accumulated doses greater than the limits was as follows:

- five in excess of the quarterly limit,
- three in excess of the annual whole body limit,
- one in excess of the annual extremity limit,
- one in excess of the annual public limit,
- one under investigation.

A dose which exceeds a regulatory limit does not mean that an injury has occurred, only that the potential risk of harm has increased. Immediate or short-term injury requires a very high dose and this is a very rare occurrence in Canada. An example of the latter occured a number of years ago when a careless radiographer received radiation burns on his fingers from touching a radioactive source.

Studies that have been carried out on nuclear reactor workers show no excess incidence of diseases, including cancer. However, studies of miners in Ontario have shown a significant excess of lung cancers among uranium miners. This has been ascribed to exposure to high levels of radon decay products in the early days of uranium mining. This excess is expected to eventually disappear at the current low levels of exposure.

Another important criterion of success in regulation is the prevention of the occurrence of accidents at nuclear facilities, which could result in radiation exposure of the public. Nuclear reactors are of special concern because of their potential for accidents resulting in the release of

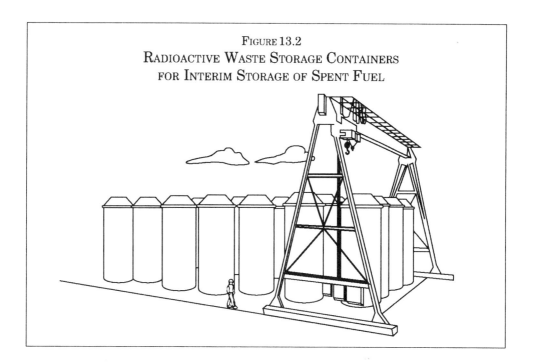

FIGURE 13.2
RADIOACTIVE WASTE STORAGE CONTAINERS
FOR INTERIM STORAGE OF SPENT FUEL

large quantities of radioactive material. There has never been a nuclear reactor incident in Canada in which a member of the public received a radiation dose exceeding the regulatory limits.

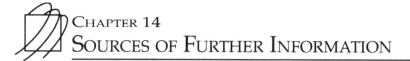

# CHAPTER 14
# SOURCES OF FURTHER INFORMATION

Many national and international organizations provide information on radiation and its effects on humans. What follows is a selected listing of sources which publish more detailed descriptions about the topics discussed in this introductory text.

## INTERNATIONAL SOURCES

### INTERNATIONAL COMMISSION ON RADIOLOGICAL PROTECTION (ICRP)

The Commission is the primary international body recommending radiation protection standards. It records in the *Annals of the ICRP* detailed reviews of the scientific basis for the recommendations made. The Annals are published by Pergammon Press, Headington Hill Hall, Oxford, OX3 OBW, United Kingdom.

### UNITED NATIONS SCIENTIFIC COMMITTEE ON THE EFFECTS OF ATOMIC RADIATION

The committee, known as UNSCEAR, is a committee established by the General Assembly of the United Nations at its tenth session in 1955. It is the main international review body on the effects of radiation. It publishes substantial reviews on the levels of radiation throughout the world from all known sources, and on the current state of knowledge about the biological effects. The last report, published in 1988, also contains a review of the large amount of information available from many parts of the world on the levels of radioactivity in the environment after the Chernobyl accident. It can be obtained from bookstores or from the United Nations, Sales Section, New York, N.Y.

### OTHER UNITED NATIONS AGENCIES

The main source is the International Atomic Energy Agency (IAEA) in Vienna, Austria, which produces numerous reports on all aspects of the peaceful uses of nuclear technology including many describing recommended safe practices. It is responsible for indexing and abstracting data pertaining to nuclear sciences and radiation protection in the International Nuclear Information System (INIS). IAEA publications may be obtained from the Division of Publications, International Atomic Energy Agency, Wagramerstrasse 5, P.O. Box 100, A-1400 Vienna, Austria, or from UNIPUB, P.O. Box 433 Murray Hill Station, New York, N.Y., 10157, U.S.A.

The World Health Organization (WHO), the International Labour Organization (ILO), United Nation Environment Program and the Food and Agricultural Organization (FAO) also publish information on radiation protection.

There are many other sources of information, particularly from individual countries in Europe, the European Commission and the U.S.A. Much of the information contained in these publications is highly detailed scientific material for the specialist. It is advisable to ask your local library to obtain these documents for examination before you purchase.

A booklet similar to this one but containing United Kingdom data was prepared by the National Radiological Protection Board (NRPB) and is available from Her Majesty's Stationery Office, Publications Centre, P.O. Box 276, London, SW8 5DT, U.K.

Many reports on radiological safety are available from the NRPB. The address is National Radiological Protection Board, Chilton, Didcot, Oxon, OX11 0RQ, U. K.

## CANADIAN SOURCES

### GOVERNMENT SOURCES

The Atomic Energy Control Board publishes documents on the regulation of the nuclear industry and on safety matters. These may be obtained free of charge from the Atomic Energy Control Board, P.O. Box 1046, Ottawa, Ontario, K1P 5S9.

An annual catalogue is published which lists all Board publications available to the public. Documents may be ordered by fax 613-992-2915, telephone 613-995-5894 or 1-800-668-5284, or letter.

Health Canada conducts a radiological surveillance program to determine levels of environmental activity in Canada and assess the resulting population exposures. An annual report of these activities is published and may be obtained by writing to the Communications Branch, Health Canada, 19th Floor, Jeanne Mance Building, Ottawa, Ontario, K1A 0K9. From time to time the department issues interpretative notes in the form of departmental documents and papers for scientific journals. Reprints of these documents are available.

Atomic Energy of Canada Limited (AECL) is the crown corporation having responsibility for research in nuclear sciences and engineering. It publishes annually numerous documents on many matters pertaining to the peaceful uses of nuclear technology. A catalogue of these documents is issued. This may be obtained by writing to Atomic Energy of Canada Limited, Chalk River, Ontario, K0J 1J0.

Environment Canada, the Department of Fisheries and Oceans, the National Research Council and other federal departments issue reports from time to time on specialized topics.

Departments of most provincial governments also prepare and publish information on nuclear matters. These may be obtained from provincial government publication sales offices.

Public utilities having nuclear generating stations (Ontario, Quebec and New Brunswick) publish annual reports of their operations and of the levels of radionuclides in water, air and foodstuffs sampled around their reactors.

Addresses from which information may be obtained are:

Director, Public Affairs
New Brunswick Power Corporation
Box 2000,
Fredericton, New Brunswick,
E3B 4X1

Corporate & Public Affairs
Ontario Hydro
700 University Avenue,
Toronto, Ontario,
M5G 1X6

Directeur-adjoint
Gestion du nucléaire
Hydro-Québec
4900, boul. Bécancour
Bécancour (Québec)
G0X 1GO

## NON-GOVERNMENT SOURCES

The Canadian Nuclear Association (CNA) is the organization representing Canadian nuclear industries. It holds workshops and seminars and issues reports on all aspects of the industry. An annual meeting is held as well as smaller meetings throughout the year to review specialized topics. Information may be obtained from the Canadian Nuclear Association, 144 Front Street West, Suite 725, Toronto, Ontario, M5J 2G7. Telephone 1-800-387-4477

The Canadian Radiation Protection Association (CRPA) is the scientific body to which many Canadians engaged in all aspects of radiological safety belong. It holds an annual meeting and publishes a newsletter. Information may be obtained from The Secretariat, 318 Lyon Street, Ottawa, Ontario, K1R 5W6.

Several federal and provincial commissions have held public hearings on different aspects of nuclear energy in various provinces, notably Ontario, Saskatchewan and British Columbia. The reports of these commissions contain much useful information. Briefs from groups opposed to nuclear technology and their views are documented in commission reports.

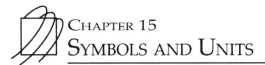

# CHAPTER 15
# SYMBOLS AND UNITS

## HISTORICAL UNITS

All our daily activities involve quantities, the distance we walk or drive, the volume of goods we buy or sell, even the amount we weigh. A quantity has two parts – a number and a unit. To say we drive at 60 has no meaning unless we also state the unit, e.g. 60 kilometres per hour or 60 miles per hour.

Whatever is convenient and makes sense will serve as a unit as long as there is general agreement on its use. When, in the bible, God told Noah to build an ark 300 cubits long, this was a unit Noah understood. The cubit is the distance between the elbow and the fingertip. It is about 51 cm and is a convenient measuring unit for a carpenter. An obvious disadvantage of this unit is that it varies with the size of the carpenter. Other parts of the body also make useful units; the hand, measuring about 10 cm across, is one such unit still used today to measure the height of horses.

The fathom, now defined as exactly six feet, was once the distance between the fingertips with arms outstretched. Sailors have used this unit to measure the depth of water for centuries. Like sailors, many tradesmen developed their own set of units, often with picturesque names. The tod, the wey and the ell of the wool trade, the cord of the woodsman and the furlong (or length of furrow ploughed by oxen before they needed a rest), are but a few examples.

Adoption of units in this way in different countries led to a bewildering number of units. In 1791 the French Academy simplified and standardized units by introducing the metric system. In English-speaking countries this system was generally adopted by scientists, but not by engineers and others. This resulted in an increased number of units in use in these countries. Confusion grew when the United Kingdom changed the sizes of some of its units but kept the old names. The Americans retained both the size and the names so that, for example, a gallon in the United Kingdom and Canada is different from a gallon in the United States.

The General Conference of Weights and Measures is an international body founded nearly 100 years ago to promote uniform units of measurement. It met in

1960 and agreed on a system based on metric measures – the Système International d'Unités or SI. This system has been adopted by all western countries except the United States. It was introduced in Canada about 20 years ago. SI units are not based on common human experience but are highly structured and rigidly defined on principles of physics and chemistry.

## RADIATION UNITS

When engineers or scientists introduce something new and the quantity of it is identified in unfamiliar units, people have no standards with which to judge whether it is big or small. This happened in Canada when SI units were introduced and reporting of temperatures was changed to Celsius from Fahrenheit. Older Canadians knew how cold it felt at ten below zero on the Fahrenheit scale but had no sense of the temperature represented by 23 below zero on the Celsius scale. Such is the case with radioactivity and the ionizing radiation it emits. To add to the

difficulty, the official radiation protection measurement units were changed in the 1970s to correspond to the new SI system. Radioactivity, radiation and radiation dose, however, are part of life and if they are to be understood this lack of familiarity has to be overcome and knowledge of units acquired. The accompanying table gives the official names of three SI units currently used in radiation protection and the corresponding older units still being used in some parts of North America. For radiation protection purposes the sievert is of most importance.

The SI unit for the activity of a radioactive source is the becquerel (abbreviation Bq). The corresponding old unit of activity is the curie (Ci). These are measures of the rate at which the atoms of the radioactive source disintegrate.

The gray (abbreviation Gy) is the SI unit of absorbed dose. This unit is used to measure the amount of radiation energy absorbed by a kilogram of tissue or other matter. The rad is the corresponding unit in the old system.

| UNITS USED IN RADIATION PROTECTION | | |
|---|---|---|
| | **SI UNITS** | **OLD UNITS** |
| Absorbed dose | gray (Gy) | rad = 0.01 Gy<br>= 10mGy |
| Equivalent dose<br>Effective dose | sievert (Sv) | rem = 0.01 Sv<br>= 10 mSv |
| Activity of radioactive substance | becquerel (Bq) | curie (Ci) = $3.7 \times 10^{10}$ Bq<br>= 37 GBq |

The harmful effects of a certain amount of radiation depends not only on the absorbed dose in the tissues and bodies of living things, but also on the type of radiation being absorbed and the body organs being exposed. For example, a gray of alpha radiation received by the lungs has more biological effect than a gray of gamma radiation or x-rays received by the thyroid. Another unit is therefore needed in radiation protection to take account of the type of radiation and the organ exposed and so permit the addition of the harmful effects of exposure to all kinds of radiation. This unit is the sievert (abbreviation Sv). In the old system the corresponding unit is the rem. The dose to a person in sieverts is known as the 'effective dose' (throughout this document 'dose' is used for effective dose). The sievert is the most important and commonly used unit in radiation protection because it is the unit that is related to the harmful effects of radiation. To relate becquerels to grays or sieverts is complex and well beyond the scope of this book.

Although the names of these radiation units are also the names of individual persons, they are not spelled with a capital first letter. However, the abbreviations are capitalized. Scientifically the units are never used in plural form, only singular. Plurals are, however, sometimes used in day to day writing.

SYMBOLS IN RADIATION PROTECTION

Symbols are used extensively in radiation protection. The elements are usually represented by symbols, for example C for carbon, Ba for Barium, and Pb for lead. It is usual to indicate the mass number and the atomic number of a particular nuclide by a superscript and subscript thus: carbon-14 by $^{14}_{6}C$, barium-140 by $^{140}_{56}Ba$, and lead-210 by $^{210}_{82}Pb$. The smaller atomic number is frequently omitted.

| COMMON SYMBOLS USED IN RADIATION PROTECTION | |
|---|---|
| SYMBOL | TERM |
| α | alpha particle |
| β | beta particle |
| γ | gamma ray |
| e | electron |
| p | proton |
| n | neutron |
| eV | electron volt |
| A | mass number |
| Bq | becquerel |
| Gy | gray |
| Sv | sievert |
| E | effective dose |
| person·Sv | person sievert |
| Z | atomic number |
| $t_{1/2}$ | half life |

## SI Prefixes

The SI system is very useful when dealing with very large or very small numbers. In both cases, when writing out the numbers, many zeros may be needed, e.g. 140 000 000 000. Note that spaces are used to separate the thousands rather than commas. This is normal SI practice, as the comma is the symbol for a decimal point in Europe. Large numbers such as that illustrated are inconvenient. It is difficult to compare numbers expressed this way because the zeros can be confusing.

Using powers of ten is a useful technique. The symbol $10^3$ means ten multiplied by itself three times or $10 \times 10 \times 10 = 1000$. The symbol $10^{-3}$ is 1 divided by 1000 or $1/(10 \times 10 \times 10) = 0.001$.

Similarly $10^6$ is one million or 10 multiplied by itself six times and $10^{-6}$ is 1 divided by 1 million. It is more convenient to use $1.4 \times 10^{11}$ than 140 000 000 000. Another simplification possible with the SI system is to use prefixes defined in the system. SI prefixes with the symbols representing them and the corresponding multiplication factors are shown in the accompanying table.

**SI Prefixes**

| Prefix | Multiplication Factor | Symbol |
|--------|----------------------|--------|
| exa | $10^{18}$ | E |
| peta | $10^{15}$ | P |
| tera | $10^{12}$ | T |
| giga | $10^9$ | G |
| mega | $10^6$ | M |
| kilo | $10^3$ | k |
| hecto | $10^2$ | h |
| deca | 10 | da |
| Base Unit | 1 | - |
| deci | $10^{-1}$ (one tenth) | d |
| centi | $10^{-2}$ (one hundredth) | c |
| milli | $10^{-3}$ (one thousandth) | m |
| micro | $10^{-6}$ (one millionth) | $\mu$ |
| nano | $10^{-9}$ | n |
| pico | $10^{-12}$ | p |
| femto | $10^{-15}$ | f |
| atto | $10^{-18}$ | a |

140 000 000 000 Bq may be written as $1.4 \times 10^{11}$ Bq or 140 GBq. It may also be written as 0.14 TBq.

The large multiplier prefixes, such as tera or exa, are useful in radiation protection because the SI unit of radioactivity, the becquerel, is small and practical quantities need big multipliers. On the other hand the dose unit, the sievert, is so big it needs small multipliers for practical quantities. Thus the Chernobyl accident in

1986 released about $10^{18}$ Bq (1 EBq) of iodine-131, which resulted in doses in Canada of about 0.0001 mSv ($10^{-7}$ Sv).

Millisieverts are practical measurement units for dose in most situations. Tera-becquerels (TBq) are usually appropriate quantities for measuring radioactive releases to the environment and millibecquerels (mBq) are appropriate for concentrations of radioactive substances, e.g. concentrations of a radionuclide in food may be expressed as mBq/kg, in water as mBq/L and in air as mBq/m³. Radioactive surface contamination might be given as kBq/m². Figure 15.1 illustrates the effects of a range of doses on individuals, dose limits and doses from various sources in both old and SI units.

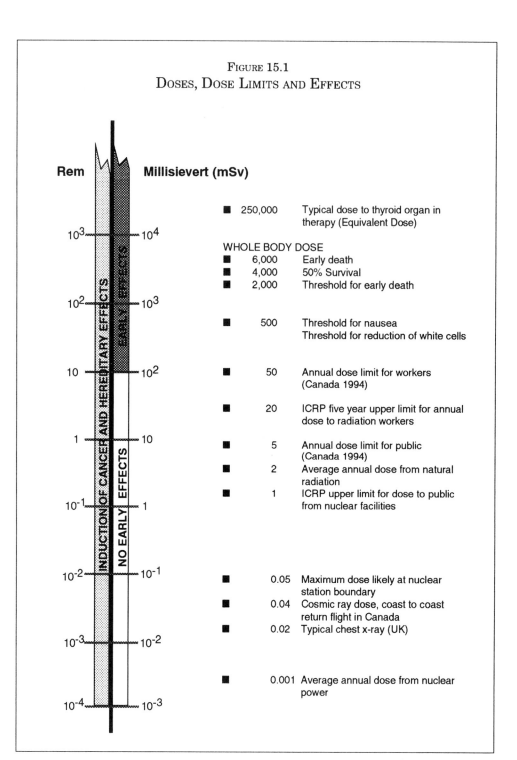

FIGURE 15.1
DOSES, DOSE LIMITS AND EFFECTS

**Rem**    **Millisievert (mSv)**

■ 250,000  Typical dose to thyroid organ in
           therapy (Equivalent Dose)

WHOLE BODY DOSE
■   6,000  Early death
■   4,000  50% Survival
■   2,000  Threshold for early death

■     500  Threshold for nausea
           Threshold for reduction of white cells

■      50  Annual dose limit for workers
           (Canada 1994)

■      20  ICRP five year upper limit for annual
           dose to radiation workers

■       5  Annual dose limit for public
           (Canada 1994)
■       2  Average annual dose from natural
           radiation
■       1  ICRP upper limit for dose to public
           from nuclear facilities

■    0.05  Maximum dose likely at nuclear
           station boundary
■    0.04  Cosmic ray dose, coast to coast
           return flight in Canada
■    0.02  Typical chest x-ray (UK)

■   0.001  Average annual dose from nuclear
           power

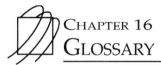

CHAPTER 16
GLOSSARY

**Absorbed dose**   Quantity of energy imparted by *ionizing radiation* to unit mass of matter such as tissue.  Unit gray, symbol Gy. 1 Gy = 1 joule per kilogram.

**Actinides**   A group of 15 *elements* with *atomic number* from that of actinium (89) to lawrencium (103) inclusive.  All are *radioactive*.  Group includes uranium, plutonium, americium and curium.

**Activity**   Attribute of an amount of *radionuclide*.  Describes the rate at which nuclear transformations occur.  Unit becquerel.  Symbol Bq.
1 Bq = 1 transformation per second.

**Alpha particle**   A particle consisting of two *protons* plus two *neutrons*.  Emitted by some *radionuclides* during their *radioactive decay* or transformation.

**Annals of the ICRP**   Documents published by the International Commission on Radiological Protection providing recommendations and guidance on radiation protection.

**Atom**   The smallest unit of an *element* that maintains the properties of the element.

**Atomic bomb**   See *nuclear weapon.*

**Atomic number**   The number of *protons* in the *nucleus* of an *atom.*  Symbol Z.

**BEIR Committee**   A committee established by the U.S. Academy of Sciences to study and report on the biological effects of ionizing radiation.

**Becquerel**   See *activity.*

**Beta particle**   An *electron* emitted from the *nucleus* of a *radionuclide.*  When its electric charge is positive the beta particle is called a *positron.*

**CANDU reactor**   Acronym for Canadian Deuterium Uranium reactor.  A reactor which uses deuterium oxide (heavy water) as moderator and coolant. The fuel is uranium oxide. The reactor has an array of pressure tubes housing the fuel, contained within a low-pressure moderator tank.

**Chromosomes**   Rod-shaped bodies found in the *nucleus* of every body cell. They contain the *genes,* or hereditary elements.  Human beings possess 23 pairs.

**Collective dose**   Frequently used for *collective effective dose.*

**Collective effective dose**   The sum of all the individual effective doses in an exposed population.  Unit person sievert, symbol person·Sv.  Frequently abbreviated to collective dose.

**Cosmic rays**   High energy *ionizing radiations* from outer space.  Complex composition at the surface of the earth.

**Cosmogenic**   Radioactive materials produced by cosmic radiation interacting with elements in the upper atmosphere.

**Decay**   The process of spontaneous transformation of a *radionuclide.*  The decrease in the *activity* of a *radioactive* substance.

**Decay product**   A *nuclide* or *radionuclide* produced by *decay.*  It may be formed directly from a radionuclide or as a result of a series of successive decays through several radionuclides.

**Disposal**   In relation to *radioactive waste,* dispersal or emplacement in any medium without the intention of retrieval.

**Depleted uranium**   Uranium in which the content of the *isotope* uranium-235 has been decreased.  Refers to a decrease below the natural value of 0.7% by weight.

**DNA**   Deoxyribonucleic acid.  The compound that controls the structure and function of cells and is the material of inheritance.

**Dose**   General term for quantity of radiation received.  See *absorbed dose, equivalent dose, effective dose, collective effective dose,* and *genetically significant dose.*  Frequently used for effective dose.

**Dosimeter**   A device for measuring radiation dose.  A personal dosimeter is a device for estimating the *effective dose* to a person by measuring the dose at a place on the body of the wearer.

**Effective dose**   The quantity obtained by multiplying the *equivalent doses* to various tissues and organs by the tissue weighting factor appropriate to each and summing the products.  Unit sievert, symbol Sv.  Tissue weighting factors are tabulated in the text.  Frequently abbreviated to dose.

**Electrical interaction**   A force of repulsion acting between electric charges of like sign and a force of attraction acting between electric charges of unlike sign.

**Electric field strength**   A measure of the intensity of an electric field.  Unit volt per metre, symbol $Vm^{-1}$.

**Electromagnetic spectrum**   All electromagnetic radiations displayed as a continuum in order of increasing frequency or decreasing wavelength.

**Electromagnetic radiation**   Radiation that can be considered as a wave of electric and magnetic energy travelling through a vacuum or a material. Examples are *x-rays, gamma rays, ultraviolet radiation, light, infrared radiation,* and *radiofrequency radiation.*

**Electron**   An elementary particle with a low mass, 1/1836 that of a proton, and with unit negative electric charge. Positively charged electrons, called positrons, also exist. See also *beta particle.*

**Electron volt**   Unit of energy employed in radiation physics. Equal to the energy gained by an electron is passing through a potential difference of 1 volt. Symbol eV.
1 eV = 1.6 x $10^{-19}$ joule approximately.

**Element**   A substance with *atoms* all of the same *atomic number.*

**Enriched uranium**   Uranium in which the content of the *isotope* uranium-235 has been increased above its natural value of 0.7% by weight.

**Equivalent dose**   The quantity obtained by multiplying the *absorbed dose* by a radiation weighting factor to allow for the different effectiveness of the various *ionizing radiations* in causing harm to tissue. Unit sievert, symbol Sv. The weighting factor for gamma rays, x-rays and beta particles is 1, but for alpha particles 20.

**Erythema**   Reddening of the skin caused by dilation of blood vessels.

**Excitation**   A process by which *radiation* imparts energy to an *atom* or *molecule* without causing *ionization.* The energy is dissipated as heat in tissue; may also cause chemical changes.

**Fallout**   Usually refers to *radionuclides* produced by *nuclear weapons* and transferred from the atmosphere to earth. Also refers to the transfer of *radionuclides* from atmosphere to earth e.g. from a gaseous plume of radioactive material from an accident.

**Fast neutrons**   Conventionally, *neutrons* with energies in excess of 0.1MeV. Corresponding velocity of about 4 x $10^6$ metres per second.

**Fission**   Nuclear fission. A process in which a *nucleus* splits into two or more nuclei and energy is released. Frequently refers to the splitting of a nucleus of uranium-235 into two approximately equal parts by a *thermal neutron* with emission of other neutrons.

**Free radical**   A grouping of *atoms* that normally exists in combination with other atoms, but can sometimes exist independently. Generally very reactive in a chemical sense.

**Frequency**   The number of complete cycles of an electromagnetic wave in a second. Unit hertz, symbol Hz. 1 Hz = 1 cycle per second.

**Fusion**   Thermonuclear fusion. A process in which two or more light *nuclei* combine to form a heavier nucleus and energy is released. Believed to be the source of energy of the sun.

**Gamma ray**   A discrete quantity of electromagnetic energy, without mass or charge. Emitted from the nucleus of certain *radionuclides* during their *radioactive decay*; cf. *x-ray*.

**Geiger tube**   A glass or metal envelope containing a gas at low pressure and two electrodes. *Ionizing radiation* causes discharges, which are registered as electric pulses in a counter. The number of pulses per second is related to the intensity of ionizing radiation.

**Genes**   The biological units of heredity. They are arranged along the length of *chromosomes*.

**Genetically significant dose**   The radiation dose to the reproductive organs prior to the conception of children. Unit sievert, symbol Sv (the unit of *equivalent dose*).

**Gray**   See *absorbed dose*.

**Half-life**   The time taken for the *activity* of a *radionuclide* to lose half its value by *decay*. Symbol $t_{1/2}$.

**Heavy water**   Deuterium oxide; water in which the common form of hydrogen atoms $_1^1 H$ are replaced by $_2^1 H$ atoms.

**Infrared radiation**   *Electromagnetic radiation* capable of producing the sensation of heat and found between *light* and *radiofrequency radiations* in the *electromagnetic spectrum*.

**Intervention levels**   Levels of dose rate in public places or activity levels in foods at which pre-determined actions are taken to reduce radiation doses to individuals or groups.

**Ion**   Electrically charged *atom*, grouping of atoms or subatomic particle.

**Ion Pair**   The electron and positively charged *ion* produced when *ionizing radiation* interacts with an atom or molecule.

**Ionization**   The process by which a neutral *atom* or *molecule* acquires or loses an electric charge. The production of *ions*.

**Ionizing radiation**   *Radiation* that produces *ionization* in matter. Examples are *alpha particles, beta particles, gamma rays. x-rays*, and *neutrons*.

**Isotope**   *Nuclides* with the same number of *protons* but different numbers of *neutrons*. Not a synonym for nuclide.

**keV**   A unit of measurement of energy. One thousand *electron volts*. The energy of radiation emitted in the radioactive decay of a radionuclide is usually measured in keV or *MeV*.

---

**Laser** (Light amplification by stimulated emission of radiation) Device which amplifies light and usually produces an extremely narrow, intense beam of light of a single wavelength.

**Light** *Electromagnetic radiation* capable of producing the sensation of vision and found between *ultraviolet* and *infrared radiations* in the *electromagnetic spectrum.*

**Mass number** The number of *protons* plus *neutrons* in the *nucleus* of an *atom.* Symbol A.

**MeV** A unit of measurement of energy. One million *electron volts.* The energy of radiation emitted in the radioactive decay of a radionuclide is usually measured in MeV or *keV.*

**Modelling** In relation to the *disposal* of *radioactive waste,* describing in quantitative terms the physical processes that influence the movement of *radionuclides* through a medium.

**Moderator** A material used in *nuclear reactors* to reduce the energy and speed of the *neutrons* produced as a result of *fission.*

**Molecule** The smallest portion of a pure substance that can exist by itself and retain the properties of the substance.

**Mutation** A chemical change in the DNA in the *nucleus of a cell.* Mutations in sperm or egg cells or their precursors may lead to inherited effects in offspring. Mutations in body cells may lead to effects in the individual.

**Neutron** A sub-atomic particle with unit atomic mass approximately and no electric charge.

**Non-ionizing radiation** *Radiation* that does not produce *ionization* in matter. Examples are *ultraviolet radiation, light, infrared radiation,* and *radiofrequency radiation.*

**Nuclear power** Power obtained from the operation of a *nuclear reactor.* Refers in the text to electric power.

**Nuclear power industry** The industry associated with the production of *nuclear power;* in Canada the mining and milling of uranium, the preparation of fuel for *nuclear reactors,* the operation of reactors, and the management of *radioactive wastes* from reactors.

**Nuclear reactor** A device in which nuclear *fission* can be sustained in a self-supporting chain reaction involving *neutrons.* In thermal reactors, fission is brought about by *thermal neutrons,* in fast reactors by *fast neutrons.*

**Nuclear weapon** Explosive device deriving its power from *fission* or *fusion* of *nuclei,* or from both.

**Nucleus** The core of an *atom*, occupying little of the volume, containing most of the mass, and bearing positive electric charge.

**Nucleus of cell** The controlling centre of the basic unit of tissue. Contains the important material *DNA*.

**Nuclide** A species of *atom* characterised by the number of *protons* and *neutrons* and, in some cases, by the energy state of the *nucleus*.

**Order of magnitude** Quantity given to the nearest power of ten. A factor of ten.

**Person sievert** See *collective effective dose*.

**Photon** The smallest unit (quantum) of *electromagnetic radiation* that can exist.

**Positron** See *beta particle*.

**Pressurized Water Reactor (PWR)** A *thermal reactor* using water as both a *moderator* and coolant. Uses *enriched uranium* oxide fuel.

**Probability** The mathematical chance that a given event will occur.

**Proton** An elementary particle with unit atomic mass approximately and unit positive electric charge.

**Radiation** Energy in the form of waves or particles. Frequently used for *ionizing radiation* in the text except when it is necessary to avoid confusion with *non-ionizing radiation*.

**Radioactive** Possessing the property of *radioactivity*.

**Radioactive waste** Apparently useless material containing *radionuclides*. Frequently categorized, in the *nuclear power industry*, according to *activity* content or *half-life*.

**Radioactivity** The property of *radionuclides* of spontaneously emitting *ionizing radiation*.

**Radiobiology** The study of the effects of *ionizing radiation* on living things.

**Radioisotope** Radioactive atoms with the same *Atomic Number* but a different *Mass Number*.

**Radiological protection** The science and practice of limiting the harm to human beings from *radiation*.

**Radionuclide** An unstable *nuclide* that emits *ionizing radiation*.

**Radon daughter products** An obsolescent term. See *radon decay products*.

**Radon decay products**   Radionuclides in the decay chain starting with radon-222. The radionuclides are attached in varying proportions to dust particles. Sometimes also known as *radon daughter products* or *radon progeny.*

**Radon progeny**   See *radon decay products.*

**Reactor Safety**   The technology, practices and procedures devoted to the prevention of reactor accidents.

**Regulating System**   The system which controls the power output of a reactor in normal conditions.

**Risk**   The *probability* of injury, harm or damage.

**Risk factor**   The *probability* of cancer and leukaemia or hereditary damage per unit *dose equivalent*. Usually refers to fatal malignant diseases and serious hereditary damage. Unit $Sv^{-1}$.

**Sievert**   See *effective dose.*

**Special Safety Systems**   Systems installed on a reactor to prevent unregulated power increases and to maintain the barriers designed to prevent the release of radioactive material from the reactor.

**Stable**   As applied to an atom means that the atom does not undergo radioactive decay or transformation.

**Thermal neutrons**   *Neutrons* that have been slowed to the degree that they have the same average thermal energy as the *atoms* or *molecules* through which they are passing. The average energy of neutrons at ordinary temperatures is about 0.025 eV, corresponding to an average velocity of $2.2 \times 10^3$ metres per second.

**Thermal reactor**   See *nuclear reactor.*

**Thermoluminescent dosimeter (Abbreviation TLD)**   A dosimeter which uses thermoluminescent material. This is a material which having been exposed to ionizing radiation releases light, in proportion to the absorbed dose, when heated.

**Threshold Dose**   The radiation dose below which no effect is observed in an individual or group of individual humans or other biological species when exposed to the radiation.

**Transuranic**   Artificially produced radioactive elements with a higher *atomic number* than uranium.

**Ultraviolet radiation**   A type of *electromagnetic radiation* found between *x-rays* and *light* in the *electromagnetic spectrum.*

**Uranium**   A naturally occurring radioactive element. Contains 99.282 % uranium-238, 0.712 % uranium-235 and 0.006 % uranium-234 by weight.

**Waste management**  The control of *radioactive waste* from creation to *disposal.*

**Wavelength**  The distance between successive crests of an electromagnetic wave passing through a given material. Unit metre, symbol m.

**WLM**  See *Working Level Month*

**Working level**  A measure of concentration of airborne contamination of short-lived radionuclides from the decay chain starting with radon-222 and ending with but not including lead-210. One WL is that concentration of short-lived radon decay products which has a potential alpha energy release of 0.004 joules ($1.3 \times 10^5$ MeV) per litre of air.

**Working level month**  A measure of exposure to airborne contamination from the short-lived radionuclides of radon-222. Symbol WLM.  Exposure to 1 *working level* for one month (170 hours).

**X-ray**  A discrete quantity of electromagnetic energy. Emitted when charged particles such as electrons are stopped by a target material, as happens in an x-ray machine ; may also be emitted from an atom when orbital electrons are displaced during radioactive decay, cf. *gamma ray.* Used in this text and colloquially to describe the film record (radiograph) of a patient's exposure to x-rays in making medical diagnoses.